Young Children in Family Therapy

Young Children in Family Therapy

by

Joan J. Zilbach, M.D.

With contributions by

Sharon Gordetsky, Ph.D.

and

David Brown, M.D.

BRUNNER/MAZEL, Publishers • New York

Library of Congress Cataloging in Publication Data

Zilbach, Joan J., 1927-
    Young children in family therapy.

    Bibliography: p. 169
    Includes index.
    1. Family psychotherapy.   2. Child psychotherapy.
3. Parent and child.   I. Gordetsky, Sharon.
II. Brown, David (David Stuart)   III. Title.
RC488.5.Z55   1985   616.89'156   85-16619
ISBN 0-87630-374-2

Published by
BRUNNER/MAZEL, INC.
19 Union Square West
New York, New York 10003

To my family, Marc, Lise, Diana, Susana, Alan, and Sandi – as we lived together you taught me most of what I know about families. And to my professional family – my colleagues Sharon, Carol and Ernie – as we learned together over many years these ideas came from all of us.

Foreword

This is a most timely volume for all therapists. Joan Zilbach has long been aware of the importance of including young children in the treatment of their families and has done so. We were privileged to include an original article of hers (Zilbach et al., 1972, The Role of the Young Child in Family Therapy) in a collection of seminal papers we edited in 1972 on family and group therapy. Through the succeeding years many family therapists have not heeded her counsel. It was too easy for many of us to find reasons to exclude the young child – and certainly if the child was not the identified client.

In this volume Dr. Zilbach traces the history of the young child in family therapy most carefully and dispassionately. Recent trends in the fields of child and family therapy indicate that Dr. Zilbach's persistent interest in why and how to work with the young child in therapy has now arrived. For example, we at the Jewish Board of Family and Children's Services are ready for it. We have been reorganizing our previously separate advanced child and family training programs into a single program that has begun to teach from a common integrated understanding of individual as well as family development and treatment. We feel this book is important enough to warrant adoption as a text for our advanced integrated program as well as for our basic inservice training. It is equally important for those who wish to focus on child therapy (which has been changing to employ more family therapy and family assessment), as well as those who are more centered in family therapy.

There is an interesting parallel between professionals' resistance to work with the young child within his or her family and among those professionals who deal with the clinical significance of sex in their marital therapy cases.

Although, on a theoretical level, everyone acknowledges the importance of both issues, large numbers of clinicians continue to avoid these areas in their practice.

Dr. Zilbach deals exquisitely with our colleagues' reasons and rationalizations for excluding the child by gently pointing out how to read children's contributions, how to handle the situation in vivo, what materials to have available and how to free ourselves to join in play. How to deal with resistances of parents and children is also admirably explicated. The presentation to the reader is so sensitive and nonjudgmental that it causes one to say to oneself, "Of course, now I can try working with young kids. I wonder why I was reluctant to, up to now." Dr. Zilbach explains that she set out to write a cookbook to tell us how to proceed with the young child. It is a cookbook in the best sense because she frees us to use our own creativity. It is easy to follow the outline she draws for us – even how to make minor changes in the office that may be necessary to adapt it to include space for the young child. I felt lovingly guided by an experienced colleague. It is rare for a teacher in our mental health field to be able to teach so well through the written word.

This book calls us back to earlier family therapy traditions, ones that had become lost to many family therapists. Although addressed largely to family and marital therapists, this volume is also a call for child therapists to extend their work with the young child's family. For example, Dr. Zilbach describes some cases of a child designated by the parent as not needing to come to sessions because he or she was "normal." When the child participated at the therapist's request the child quickly revealed significant behavioral problems and/or psychopathology that had been denied by the parents. Sometimes such a child bore intergenerational stigmata. In other situations the child was not necessarily symptomatic but provided information in his or her play or even verbally that made clear important family system dynamics that had not been apparent previously.

The young child is indeed an important part of all family systems. Yes, the time has arrived for this book.

Clifford J. Sager, M.D.
Director of Family Psychiatry,
Jewish Board of Family and Children's Services;
Clinical Professor of Psychiatry,
New York Hospital-Cornell Medical Center

Contents

Foreword by Clifford J. Sager, M.D....vii

Acknowledgments...xi

1. Introduction..1

2. Play in Family Therapy: "Go Away and Play – You May Stay
   If You Talk"..11

3. In Search of Children and Play: Through the Family
   Therapy Literature...25

4. Critical Functions of Young Children in Family Therapy.............49

5. Illustrated Critical Functions..71
   with Sharon Gordetsky

6. A Family in Treatment: Selected Themes and Drawings..............89
   with Sharon Gordetsky and David Brown

7. How-To: Some Specifics on Young Children in
   Family Therapy...125

8. Finale: "I'll Be Glad to See All of You – Including the
   Little Ones"...159

Epilogue: Hopes..165

Specific References to Young Children in Family Therapy..............167

Bibliography...169

Index..175

Acknowledgments

This book developed over many years. The general outline and some details of this development can be found in the Introduction. However, here I would like to be more specific in my acknowledgments. The book is dedicated to my immediate family not only because of their years of teaching me but also because they lived through the time of struggle in the years of writing and finally producing this book. They were always encouraging, supportive, and patient.

As we began our work with families at the Judge Baker Guidance Center in the mid-1950s, Carol Gass and Ernest Bergel were brave and persistent as we encountered many internal and external difficulties. Our discussion sessions were a regularly important part of my clinical and personal development – enjoyable and rewarding as we started together to think "family as a unit," which eventually became the core of the ideas and practices described and discussed in this book.

In more recent years, Sharon Gordetsky has been an invaluable colleague. From our work together, and with the assistance of David Brown, Chapters 5 and 6 were created.

And lastly, I am deeply and personally indebted to Sue Jensen and Clinton Phillips for our family work. Without that this book would not have been finished.

Cynthia Stead provided encouragement and excellent technical typing.

The families that provided the clinical material will not recognize themselves. But their contributions were immeasurably invaluable.
Thank you.

J. J. Zilbach
Brookline, MA
1985

Young Children
in
Family Therapy

1

Introduction

Alice was beginning to get very tired of sitting by her sister on the bank and of having nothing to do: once or twice she had peeped into the book her sister was reading, but it had no pictures or conversations in it. "And what is the use of a book," thought Alice, "without pictures or conversations?"

So she was considering, in her own mind (as well as she could, for the hot day made her feel very sleepy and stupid), whether the pleasure of making a daisy-chain would be worth the trouble of getting up and picking the daisies, when suddenly a white rabbit with pink eyes ran close by her.

– Carroll (1865) 1941, p. 5

The author of this book feels the way Alice did on that sunny day. The reader may have the choice between making a daisy-chain and reading this book. It is unlikely that the white rabbit will come by, but I do hope that something will happen to the reader. Perhaps not quite as pleasant or dramatic as happened to Alice in *Alice in Wonderland* or *Through the Looking Glass*, but something . . .

This book contains both pictures and conversations, but I hope this will not deter the reader from following any white rabbits with pink eyes that may appear. For, as we know, some of our finest insights appear when, a little less alert than usual, we allow our thoughts to "stray" and follow unfamiliar paths.

Some years ago, after I had finished my training in child and adult psychiatry, I joined a research project on delinquency. Shortly thereafter, I was asked to become a consultant to an action program that attempted to work with members of inner-city female gangs out of the clinic, in the neighborhood, on the street. This was "street corner work" and the therapists were called "detached workers" – perhaps to avoid the term "street workers"! Out on the street, with no office walls available, our "patients," the young female gang members, did not know about the existing therapeutic rules of the day: that therapists spoke only to their patients and not to their families! The "street workers," consultants, and others soon knew about, had met, and were involved with whole families rather than with isolated, single, gang members.

In 1955, when the field of family therapy was in its infancy, I began to wonder and worry about families. When I returned to my professional home-base, the Judge Baker Guidance Center in Boston, to extend the work I had begun with families out in the community, I took the usual educational approach to learning. I read what little was available on working with whole families in treatment and wondered what others were doing.

Training in family therapy did not exist in my early years in psychiatry. But over and above that, it is important to note that child and adult psychiatry were, and still are, very separate endeavors when it comes to acquiring knowledge and skill. The practice of family therapy involves extensive knowledge of both children and adults and could act as a bridge with child psychiatry, in particular. This has not occurred in any strong or systematic fashion. The nondevelopment of family therapy as a bridge was discussed extensively by McDermott and Char (1974):

> . . . [family therapy] has the potential as a new treatment modality in the 1950s, for improving not only the quality, but also the quantity of mental health care for families and their members. However, instead of becoming a vehicle through which new therapists could become skilled in dealing with children as with adults, its influence may have caused children to become *less* well served than before. (p. 422)

My initial training in adult psychiatry, similar to many others in this field, was in a state hospital. Here, after the initial history taking, the family was totally dismissed, being merely the "relatives" of the important one, the patient. Much of the time, family members were considered potential nuisances when, during carefully time-regulated brief sessions, they asked troublesome and often unanswerable questions such as: "What's wrong with him?" or "When is she going to get out?"

In child psychiatry training it was a bit different. The parents, usually the mother, had to be included in order for the therapist to see the child. But she and, occasionally, other family members were seen separately in treatment, often by practitioners of other mental health disciplines, such as social workers and psychologists. I have described these states of separateness particularly for younger readers, who may not have experienced the overt shunning and banning of whole, or parts of, families that made up my own training experience and that of others of my generation.

In a few clinical settings some work with whole families in family therapy sessions was already underway. Some of these training clinics made themselves available for learning by direct observation about this new therapeutic modality. I went with a colleague on a visit to a family therapy unit in a distant place. We were excited as we wondered and talked about what might actually happen in the family therapy session that we were going to observe in action.

When we arrived, we were greeted and ushered into a small observation room with a one-way mirror, crowded with many other eager, uninformed observers. We were familiar with direct observation rooms because we used this technique for training purposes in the children's group therapy program at our clinic. As we peered through the one-way mirror we saw a small, nondescript, grayish therapy room with a large table in the center occupying most of the space in the room. There were no other furnishings or decoration in this family therapy room. As we began our observations, the family and therapists were already seated, Father at the head of the table, Mother at the opposite end, two young school-age children on either side of the table with a therapist next to each of them. The talk was rather dreary, and the temperature in the observation room rose. At one point, I was startled to find myself dozing, and when I looked up, I saw both young children in the family therapy session also asleep. Afterwards, my colleague and I shared our disappointment and many questions about this family session. However, this experience proved fortunate since it alerted us to the heretofore unobserved and contrasting style and format in our own emerging family therapy endeavors.

In the mid-1950s, at the Judge Baker Guidance Center, we began a family therapy pilot project in which we treated whole families and gradually developed a full training program in family therapy. As part of a child guidance clinic, there was never a question about inclusion of children of all ages, even the very young, nonverbal ones, in the family treatment.

In addition, we were trained in play therapy so that there were toys in the room automatically. And, as if to add emphasis to our inclusion of play materials, one of our first families had a four-and-a-half-year-old child who spontaneously brought her own toys and crayons to the very first session she attended. This young child played happily and colored throughout this therapy session with the whole family. Development of our format at this very early stage occurred without much specific thought, emerging from generalized child guidance practice. Our visit to a family therapy session in the far-away adult "talking" clinic had allowed us to observe at a distance, and return to reflect upon and further develop our own philosophy and practice of family therapy.

By this time, the reader may be wondering about "young children." Our definition of young children might be those usually excluded from family therapy! However, to be a bit more precise, they are children younger than the age of reason or, a bit more seriously, those for whom intelligent adult verbal communication is but a small part of their repertoire. These are the children for whom play and action, rather than extensive discussion, are still most important. In chronological age this is, roughly, pre-school and younger to approximately the middle of the early elementary school years. Though the emphasis in this book is primarily on young children, at times older children will appear in a case illustration when they made such a clear statement, e.g., in a striking drawing, that it had to be included.

In the following chapters, the reader will find descriptions, pictures, and explanations about young children and family therapy. And, in addition, some attention is paid to the already existing family therapy literature, although children and play have been given little direct attention in this literature. A full coverage of the rapidly expanding family therapy literature as a whole is a task which would detract from the purposes of this book. However, although we will not discuss in any detail the many different "branches" and "brands" of family therapy that exist at this time, there are some important differences within the schools of family therapy in their orientation to young children which will be discussed in Chapter 3.

Sometimes the purpose or message of a book and other communications remains hidden until the very end when it is announced in the conclusion. I will be explicit at the outset: 1) Young children can and should be considered as part of the treatment unit in family therapy; and 2) there are some specific techniques that are useful to know when young children are included in family therapy sessions. The critical functions of young children in family therapy will be discussed in Chapter 4, and illustrated in Chapters 5 and 6. Some specific techniques will be found in Chapter 7 on "How-to." Chapter 8 and the Epilogue will reiterate the message.

This brief introduction already contains important common words and terms which will appear frequently throughout this book. But, common or frequent usage does not automatically bring about clear and specific meaning – rather it is often the reverse. For the purpose of clarity, and with the hope that the rest of the book will benefit, some familiar words and terms will be defined and discussed at the outset. Beyond the two previous explicit statements of position, there are some other basic underlying assumptions which will be explicated within the following discussion of the terms: family, family development, and family therapy.

DEFINITIONS AND DISCUSSION

Familiar

"Familiar." Have you ever noticed or put that very ordinary and common word "familiar" off by itself in order to give it some distance, and then wondered about it? A good place to start is in the dictionary:

> **Familiar** 1. originally having to do with a *family* [author's emphasis]. 2. friendly; intimate; close: as *familiar* conversation. 3. too friendly; presumptuous; unduly intimate or bold. 4. closely acquainted (with). 5. well known; common; ordinary . . . – *familiar* is applied to that which is known through constant association, and with reference to persons, suggests informality, or even presumption, such as might prevail among members of a family. (Webster, 1962)

Thus, an attempt to become familiar or to assist others with increasing their familiarity may be either friendly, intimate and close, or too friendly, presumptuous, or even bold!

This book on family therapy faces all those alternatives. Which will it be? Friendly and intimate, or presumptuous and bold, as it attempts to have the reader become familiar with and closer to young children in family therapy.

Family

> What is meant by a family? . . . the very omnipresence of the family renders it almost invisible. Because we are truly immersed in the family we rarely have to define it or describe it to one another.
>
> –Degler, 1980, p. 3

5

What is a family? We think we know the answer because all of us are from a family, and remain within a family as we grow, change and create new families. Though we know so well what a family is, there are many varying definitions in implicit use in clinical practice and in explicit use within the family therapy literature. Some of these variations arise from the language developed by a particular branch of a family therapy. Others are influenced by their origins in fields such as anthropology and sociology, with their specialized languages (Note 1).

The following definition of family works for me as a clinician, researcher, family therapist, and psychoanalyst, because it includes and emphasizes salient, observable characteristics of the family: *A family is a special kind of small, natural group in which members are related by birth, marriage, or other form which creates a home or a functional household unit.* This special natural unit includes alternative family units, operates in its household functioning with some universal characteristics, and others which vary in different cultures, times, and places (Zilbach, 1979). For our purposes, among other basic family functions, the care of children/other dependent members, in a broad sense including many aspects of development, is a basic function of all family members (Notes 2 and 3).

Family Development

The family, as just defined, is an ever-changing unit. Family changes occur over time in expectable and observable phases in the course of the family life cycle. The concept of family development encompasses this series of changes and is clearly distinguishable from the development of one family member within his or her own, individual life cycle.

The following chart outlines my stages of family development:

Table 1. Family Development: Stages of the Family Life Cycle

Gestational: Courtship and Engagement or other Introductory Variant

EARLY STAGES: Forming and Nesting

Stage I. Coupling

The family begins at the point of marriage and/or the establishment of a common household by two people.

Family Task: Independence to interdependence

Stage II. Becoming Three

The second phase in family life is initiated by the arrival and subsequent inclusion/incorporation of the first child/dependent member.

Family Task: Interdependence to incorporation of dependence

MIDDLE STAGES: Family Separation Processes

Stage III. Entrances

The third phase is signaled by the exit of a first child/dependent member from the immediate world of the family to the larger world. This occurs at the point of entrance into school or other extrafamilial environment.

Family Task: Dependence to beginning separations-partial independence

Stage IV. Expansion

This phase is marked by the entrance of the last child/dependent member of the family into the larger community.

Family Task: Continuing expansion of partial separations – independence

Stage V. Exits

This phase starts with the first complete exit of a dependent member from the family. This stage marker is achieved by the establishment of an independent household which may include marriage or another form of independent entity.

Family Task: Partial separations to first complete independence

LATE STAGES: Finishing

Stage VI. Becoming Smaller/Extended

Ultimately the moment comes for the exit of the last child/dependent member from the family. (This has been incorrectly termed the "shrunken family" or "empty nest.") It may include the beginning of grandparenthood.

Family Task: Continuing expansion of independence

Stage VII. Endings

The final years start with death of one spouse/partner and continue up to the point of death of the other partner.

Revised from Zilbach, 1968; 1979; 1982

7

This conceptualization of the family life cycle is somewhat different from others (see Carter & McGoldrick, 1980). It is based on the necessary basic family functions of the whole family unit (Zilbach, 1968; 1979; 1982). Other versions of family life cycle stages are often based on the age and stage of the children, such as birth of first child, the family with adolescents, etc. These are not truly family-as-a-unit phases. In addition, this chart encompasses a variety of family structures containing children at many ages. Thus, family therapy with young children may occur at any stage of the family life cycle, not just during the early stages as one initially might think. The family therapy cases in this book are mostly in the middle stages of the family life cycle.

Family Therapy

What is family therapy? The question more accurately stated, since currently there are many varieties of family therapy, is what are the family therapies? One universal or underlying characteristic of all forms of family therapy is that the family rather than the individual is considered *the* unit of treatment. Every family therapist has an inner image or theoretical conception of the family which molds in some fashion their practice of family treatment and, particularly, their role as therapist in family treatment. But there is little disagreement about the conception of the whole family as the unit of treatment in family therapy. That children are essential parts of the family as a whole is also indisputable.

However, in reality, the unit of family treatment in clinical practice is frequently *not* the family. Rather, the unit of family treatment is often incomplete – it is the family *without* the younger children. This book grew out of years of informal observation of this exclusion. At the same time, our experiences increased and strengthened an orientation to and belief in the importance of inclusion of younger children when treating the "whole" family.

CHAPTER NOTES

1) A good example is Parsons and Bales (1955) who are well known for their work on family theory with an emphasis on role and structure. Notice the language in their partial definition of family:

> By virtue of being a small group, the nuclear family is relatively a very simple social system, and we believe this fact to be of the greatest importance for its functioning as the agency of socialization and as personality stabilization . . . . (p. viii)

Another example is George Peter Murdock, an eminent social scientist, who wrote *Social Structure* (1949). This monumental work on social theory with elements from the fields of anthropology, sociology, and psychology melded into his attempt at a "new science of human behavior." His work emphasizes kinship organization, and the language of anthropology, in particular, is utilized. His basic definition of the family is simple:

> The family is a social group characterized by common residence, and economic cooperation, and reproduction. (p. 1)

2) This definition of the family is a household definition, i.e., an "under-the-roof" definition. This is clinically useful and also has another advantage of being the same definition used by the Census Bureau so that a family clinician can compare his sample with the population as a whole. It is not often that this is important to a family therapist but it might be, and by using such a definition, it becomes possible.

3) The differences in definitions of family by family therapists are reflections of the theoretical orientation of the definer. Compare the definition by Zilbach (see page 6) with the following by a family therapist, Phillips (1980), who had a more marked systems orientation:

> A family system is a group of individuals who are related by marriage, blood, or by adoption and who have an emotional history which continues into the future. These persons are organized, structured, and function in an interdependent fashion and thereby evidence wholeness and are obviously interdependent so that the behavior of all of the members affects each and the behavior of each member has an effect upon all the members. (p. 11)

Minuchin (1974) with his structural orientation, has a different definition:

> A family is a system that operates through transactional patterns. Repeated transactions establish patterns of how, when, and to whom to relate, and these patterns underpin the system. (p. 51)

9

2

Play in Family Therapy: "Go Away and Play— You May Stay If You Talk"

> . . . it is play that is the universal, *and that belongs to health; playing leads into group relationships;* playing can be a form of communication in psychotherapy . . .
>
> > –Winnicott, 1971a, p. 41

> *Play has been hailed as the precursor of work by many psychologists. . . . There is no difficulty in following the child's activities through their various stages; play on his own and his mother's body; play with soft toys; filling and emptying containers; construction toys; role play; games; hobbies; finally, work. . . .*
>
> > –A. Freud, 1981a, p. 131

An obvious and important, yet often overlooked reason for excluding children, particularly younger children, in family therapy, is that they are children. They will not behave or speak like adults – they play and act as children do. Children may not be willing or able to sit still in their chairs and talk for the entire, or even a minor portion of, the prescribed family treatment time. They move about and otherwise express themselves physically and motorically, in nonverbal ways which may not be comfortable to adults, parents, and "talking" therapists. Some avenues of expression may be fright-

11

ening, or even distasteful and unpleasant, to adults who have forgotten or otherwise dismissed for themselves the favorite childhood expressive tools of play and drawing. Adult talk and understanding often seem so different and far away from the movement and content of children's play.

The need for the comfortable and frequent use of "regression in the service of the ego" (Kris, 1952), is confronted early in child therapists' training. As they learn, or relearn, how to play in the course of working with children, they encounter within themselves inner obstacles, resistance to this experience as an adult. However, adult therapists who concentrate on learning the intricacies of "talking" therapies only may not experience this need in the course of their therapeutic training and subsequent work. "Regression in the service of the ego" is a powerful concept and was discussed extensively by Kris (1952) in connection with creativity and artistic production. However, its import is far-reaching and most important in our work as family therapists who include young children in therapeutic endeavors as well.

Play is child's work. But, how often is this work really valued by the adults around the child? The adults may acknowledge the play in distant and vague language, but be unable to join the concrete play action. Most often they do not regard play as serious work or with the same amount of importance as verbal or written words. When is the outcome of a child's game or puppet play spoken of with the same intensity, seriousness, and concern as the final score in an adult game of baseball, football, or other "important" tournament? A supervisor may question a family therapist, "Do you think the family is working in treatment?" But have you ever heard a teacher or supervisor ask, "Are the children in the family playing?" And then, if the answer is "no," state, "Their work is not progressing." On the contrary, the absence of play is often regarded by serious adult therapists and their supervisors as progress! When a child "talks," therapy is considered to be going well. But the knowledgeable "child-including" family therapist will disagree with this positive judgment if play is absent or minimal throughout the family sessions.

An ordinary dictionary reveals some further evidence of typical adult attitudes toward play in its definitions:

1) to engage in sport or diversion; to amuse oneself,
2) to take part in a game of skill or chance and,
3) to act in a way *not* to be taken seriously. . . .
   (Funk & Wagnall, 1980, p. 106, author's emphasis)

The last definition, "to act in a way *not* to be taken seriously," makes clear a prevailing attitude toward play. These definitions were taken from one standard dictionary but the same attitude can be found in others such as the *Webster's Deluxe Unabridged Dictionary* (Webster, 1979). It is quite prevalent! This attitude, which exists so strongly in society in general, is often also held by family therapists.

How much and what kind of attention is devoted to play? "Go play, children," is frequently a peremptory dismissal. Playtime is thought of as "time off," a "recess," "let's take a break and go to the game." These are just a few everyday confirmatory examples of the attitudes previously noted in the dictionary definitions.

Yet, adults, in their unspoken dreams and fantasies, may pleasantly remember some sunny, bright days of early childhood filled with play. As they reflect, they imagine brightly-colored mobiles floating over the crib of a newborn, then the first rattle, stuffed animals, dolls, building blocks, and on to complicated erector sets, train sets, and more. The increasing complexity in this progressive play sequence with toys also occurs in another sequence of play development in drawing from scribbles, to stick figures, and then to increasingly realistic figures made in clay, crayons, paint, and water. These are the toys and materials used by children. Adolescents and adults have their own special toys. The rapid growth of the electronic game industry attests to the continuing and expanding interest and participation by adults in play throughout an individual's lifetime.

Adults often feel freer to observe and express an interest in play when it is accompanied by obvious "learning" as in the play activities of young babies. Then, overt signs of adult interest in play are easily discerned in statements such as, "Look at baby smile – she's learning by playing with that toy!" Adult interest in the growth and development of babies is well accepted. But is play considered with as much interest as children grow older? Young children, in particular, even when they progress rapidly and "talk early," continue to need play and other nonverbal modes of expression for their successful development. Play may be recognized by parents as an important after-school, non-"educational" activity with the peers of school-age children. Sports as play may become quite important to some families. Exceptional families with adult children that continue to play either singly or together and go "public," regard these activities as their profession – their "work." The tennis Austin and Evert families, the singing Taylors, the skiing Corcorans and Mahres, the skating Howes are examples of families for whom play has become important and productive work. However, for most adults play occupies time and attention that is merely "leftover"!

13

Some professionals must overcome these attitudes since play and other kinds of fun-activities occupy such a prominent place in early child development.

Early in the history of psychoanalysis as a profession, an interest in treating children developed with play as an essential part of the treatment process. Play is an essential ingredient in the work of Klein, an early and important contributer to the development of child analysis (Klein, 1932).

Later, "play therapy" as a distinct therapeutic modality has developed along with, but separate from, child analysis. Play therapy is not to be confused with the topic of this chapter, Play in Family Therapy. Play therapy is another distinct form of psychotherapy. In a classic book in this field, *Play Therapy*, Axline (1947) defines play therapy as:

> . . . based upon the fact that play is the child's natural medium of self-expression. It is an opportunity which is given to the child to "play-out" his feelings and problems just as, in certain types of adult therapy, an individual "talks-out" his difficulties. (p. 9)

> Since play is his natural medium for self-expression, the child is given the opportunity to play out his accumulated feelings of tension, frustration, insecurity, aggression, fear, bewilderment, and confusion. (p. 16)

For our purposes, we note that play therapy has therapeutic value and that such therapists are "trained" to play with children. Family therapists bring their training about children in from other training, outside the family field. Few family training programs actually teach or even discuss playing with children in family therapy.

Another notable child therapist, D. W. Winnicott, not only included play, but was a masterful inventor of a child therapeutic game, the "Squiggle" game. Though he is best known for some important theoretical constructs such as the "holding environment" and the "good enough mother" we take particular note of him as a playful therapist and the inventor of this therapeutic game:

> In this "squiggle" game, I make some kind of impulsive line-drawing and invite the child whom I am interviewing to turn it into something, and then he makes the squiggle for me to turn into something in my turn." (p. 16) (Note 1)

Anna Freud has added important dimensions to our understanding of play with her elucidation of the concept of developmental lines:

> . . . to investigate development, it doesn't suffice [to investigate only] the past. It is equally imperative to follow each psychic element in its *forward* course until the time when it qualifies for becoming part of the mature, adult personality; to watch and describe the interaction of the various elements with each other; to study how far they help or hinder each other's advance; how they combine with each other and how they finally produce the qualities, attitudes, and abilities. . . . a sequence of developmental steps can be established for the individuals arriving at the ability to work. . . . (1981a, p. 129, author's emphasis)

We are particularly concerned with the developmental lines *from play to work*, since the various levels of play are the important building blocks which lead to the development of work competence:

> We find a similar array of factors active on the line *from play to work*. As regards to the consecutive forms of play (on the mother's body, with soft toys, with sand and water, with filling and emptying, with constructive toys, role play, games, hobbies). . . .
> Finally . . . the ego outgrows the need for immediate pleasure gain, its newly acquired way of functioning according to the reality principle changes the infantile activity of play into the all important mature capacity to work. (Freud, A., 1981b, p. 103)

In the course of formulating his psychosocial lines of development, which significantly expanded our understanding of psychosexual development, Eric Erikson did research on play (1951). In *Childhood and Society* (Erikson, 1950; 1963), he discusses play extensively. He emphasizes the interpersonal and cultural/social aspects of play as growth-promoting qualities for the young, developing child.

Sigmund Freud was also interested in the play of young children. In an early paper, "Creative Writers and Daydreaming" (Freud, 1908), he emphasized the importance of play in its relationship to creativity:

> If we could at least discover in ourselves or in people like ourselves an activity which was in some way akin to creative writing! An examination of it would then give us a hope of obtaining the beginnings of an explanation of . . . creative work. . . .

Should we not look for the first traces of imaginative activity as early in childhood? The child's best-loved and most intense occupation is with his play or games. Might we not say that every child at play behaves like a creative writer, in that he creates a world of his own, or, rather, rearranges the things of his world in a way which pleases him? It would be wrong to think that he does not take that world seriously; on the contrary, he takes his play very seriously and expends large amounts of emotion on it. The opposite of play is not what is serious, but what is real. . . . (pp. 143–144)

Readers who become interested in the relationship between play and creative activities will find this short paper intriguing.

Observations of play in young children were major sources of data for Jean Piaget in his developmental theory. His observations of his own children were reported in *The Origins of Intelligence* (1952), the *Construction of Reality in the Child* (1954), and *Play, Dreams, and Imitation in Childhood* (1951). Piaget's work is an excellent and important example of utilizing observations of play in theory development.

However, our concern in this volume is mainly therapeutic. Play as therapy for children began historically with Freud's famous case, "Little Hans" (1909). In this case, Little Hans's Father drew a picture of a giraffe and Hans added a "widdler" (penis) which his Father took to and talked about with "the Professor" (Freud). In this case the drawing and other material were carefully observed, recorded, and discussed in this case for generations of therapists to see, understand, and use in their own development of understanding of young children. The "widdler" is drawn clearly – the text tells us its meaning. (See *Standard Edition*, Vol. 10, p. 13, for a reproduction of the original picture of the giraffe and its "widdler.")

Child psychiatrists and other child diagnosticians attribute considerable importance to play activities and will ask in the course of an evaluation interview with parents, "How does the child play with his peers?" Later in the course of treatment, a child therapist may become concerned about a father-son relationship that has been minimal or absent and encourage them to "play together" at home in sports activities, e.g., "Go and throw a ball with him" (Note 1).

Play is regarded as "serious business" by family therapists who do include children in their family therapy sessions. When children are included

16

in family sessions, therapists watch carefully, join, and, through the observation of play, drawing, bodily movement, and other actions, gain further understanding of children and their families which becomes therapeutically useful. In general, the functions of play in family therapy are:

1) Direct expression and enactment of important family material, e.g., doll play of family fights, puppet enactments of divorce.
2) Reduction of anxiety, e.g., becoming absorbed in a repetitive and engrossing play activity, such as a checkers game, repetitive and simple drawings, or making simple clay objects, while other family members are discussing painful material.
3) Defense against anxiety through more passive participation, diversion, or absence, e.g., playing a radio with earplugs during a parental fight, leaving the therapy room to get paint, water, or other supplies.

These functions of play can be seen in the pictures that follow. An accompanying explanation is provided for each picture.

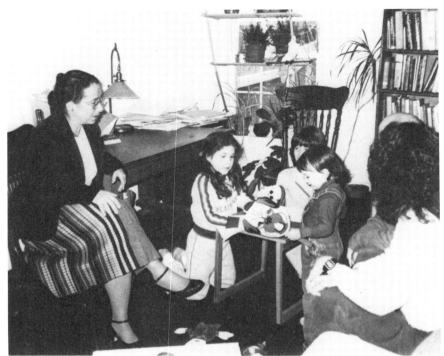

Photo 2.1

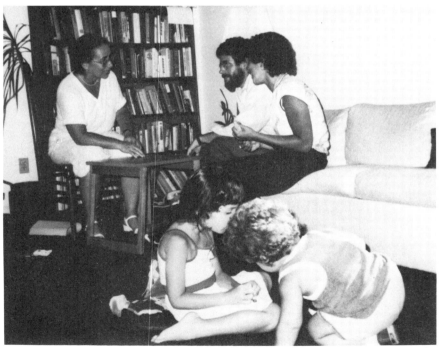

Photo 2.2

18

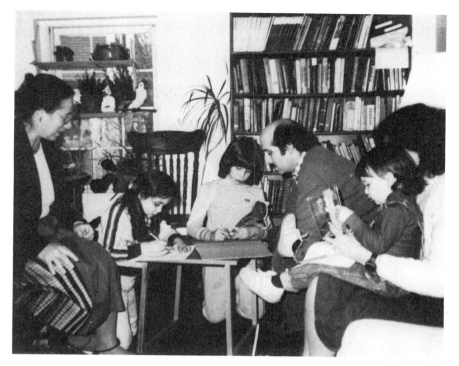

Photo 2.3

FUNCTIONS OF PLAY

Direct Enactment. The children are busily telling a "family" story using puppets. The youngest child, on the right, is playing a "mother" animal puppet character. The older two children are using hand puppets as sibling characters. The real mother, in the foreground, sits stiffly upright, uncomfortably listening to the children's "family" tale. (Photo 2.1)

Reduction of Anxiety. With increasing intensity, the parents are telling the therapists, about their children, home life, and problems. Notice the children. They have moved away from the parents on the couch and physically closer to each other, in their own space, they play on the floor. (Photo 2.2)

Passive Participation-Diversion. Triple diversion: The oldest child has called Father away from heated conversation with Mother to look at her picture. The youngest child sitting in Mother's lap had been quietly looking at a picture book, added to the diversion by asking, "What's this?" The third child, closest to the therapist called her attention to a detail of her picture. (Diversion does not require the participation of all children – one may do it very well alone!) (Photo 2.3)

All of these and other functions of play activities can be recognized easily in both family life and family therapy sessions. Play as direct expression, as defense against anxiety, and for other uses will be further described and illustrated in Chapters 4, 5, and 6.

The nondevelopment, impediments, and interference with play are as important to observe as the expression and use of play. Examples of such impediments will be described in Chapter 5.

EXCLUSION

Many family therapists only minimally recognize when, how, or why they exclude children. The exclusion may take the form of identifying only the family members to be included, as in "There is marital trouble – I will see the couple." These statements are not often followed by "I will not see the children" – this just happens! The term "exclusion" usually reflects implicit attitudes, expressed in covert statements and actions, rather than in clear, overt, and explicit attitudes. The family therapist's decision to see parents and not children can be a deliberate act of omission with a particular, therapeutic goal. Both are actions, but usually exclusion occurs by default, inattention or other unrecognized attitudes on the part of the therapist. Deliberate omission implies that considerable attention and planning has occurred.

An ability to participate in playful activities, combined with knowledge, facilitates a positive inclusion of young children in family therapy. However, gaining knowledge from lectures, articles, and even good books or plays, does not automatically overcome strongly developed adult attitudes and feelings. For many therapists, "Go outside and play" remains connected with parental disapproval and is a dismissal, as in the statement, "Go outside and get lost!" These attitudes are exemplified in the following examples:

A group of family therapy trainees were discussing their own childhood experiences with play. The seminar leader exclaimed, "Go outside and play! What does that remind you of?" Mr. A., a large, broad-shouldered, strong-looking man loudly proclaimed, "It means I was too boisterous. It was really a reprimand for disturbing my father who wanted to read and needed quiet. So, I would go outside whether I wanted to or not and look for my friends." After a pause he added, "I still play outside. I am rarely comfortable inside. I go outside and play 'trucks'." His face changed expression as he talked about his delight in adult "outside" fun – backpacking and conquering mountains. Imagine what this therapist, Mr. A., might feel "inside" a therapy room playing with a young child. It is likely that such a therapist would have great difficulty feeling comfortable "inside" unless some of this personal childhood feeling about play became available to him and was resolved with some comfort and pleasure in being "inside."

Exclusion is often based on inner reluctance or even strong aversion to playing with children:

In a discussion of techniques in family therapy, an experienced family therapist blurted out, "Play is useless." Surprised looks ringed the roomful of therapists. Mr. B. immediately corrected himself, "Oh, I mean nongoal-oriented activity – not play." He then added, in a very intellectual tone, "Well I know that play is a child's work, but. . . . " Other trainees pointed out that he was really scoffing at this notion. He answered by giving a lecture on specific details of developmental levels of child's play. At the end, when questioned again about play, he could not admit his evident underlying attitude. Child development had taught him about children's "work" and he persisted with his obvious intellectualizations. It is not likely that this therapist will be able to play comfortably even though he "knows" many details about the development of children. Exclusion will be explained away in length, breadth, and detail by therapists such as Mr. B.

The underlying attitude toward play as useless, and "nongoal-oriented" cannot be addressed easily with simple rational explanations. But, the underlying powerful affect can become evident:

In discussion of play in family therapy, trainees in family therapy were asked, "Where did you play in your house?" (i.e., childhood house). Ms. C., sitting curled up in a chair looking like a lost waif, answered, "We had no toys. We played with rocks and pebbles outside. Later on, when I could read, I sat in a chair all day, and I read, and read, and read." She recognized as she made this statement that she had felt very sad as the seminar leader talked about play. Had Ms. C.'s sadness gone unnoticed and unexpressed it might have become an inner impediment to further therapeutic play with children. Early deprivation of play action and play materials may lead to later inhibition and inability to use childhood play materials. For such therapists, children's books may be easier to use as therapeutic aids than the other play aids in the family therapy toy box. Experimentation with child materials that are comfortable for the therapist is encouraged, though always contained within therapeutic limits.

Other childhood issues may interfere as well:

> After a discussion about making a safe play space in the office for young children, Mr. D. said angrily, "This is too much fuss about nothing – safety. There is no need for any special place." In Mr. D.'s childhood he was the family's "bad boy." Often punishment consisted of being sent outside. He recalled that the special "inside" places belonged only to his "good" brothers and sisters. He was not going to deliberately make another "good-safe" place for them inside, in his own office space, his personal office! Mr. D.'s exclusion of children was based on his feelings about the favored position of his siblings in his own family of origin.

A nonrecognition of these attitudes by family therapists often promotes the exclusion of younger children, and then play is not a problem because treatment with only adults is primarily verbal. However, if therapists become aware of their attitudes, they may want to "learn" to play and later even to enjoy it!

It is not difficult to play! Most children are wonderful teachers. The baby starts this play-teaching by offering the bystander their first toy – a rattle – and laughing happily when it is returned. The baby is even more delighted when a little noise accompanies the return action. The toddler automatically, and with little hesitation, rolls her truck toward an adult, and waits and watches for more turns in this play. Children are often the initiators of play. "Draw me a face" is a natural request when a young child notices the paper and crayons in the family therapist's office. The adult worries and thinks, "How can I do that best?" Simple lines will suffice, making eyes, ears, and a nose, and may be accompanied by a question such as, "Is this face sad or happy?" and then adding the mouth in accord with the child's answer.

"I have to go" is a direct request by a younger child that a toilet trip is needed. However, this may lead to unexpected play! The toilet paper is pulled with enthusiasm and playfully rolled into a large ball. There are many opportunities for play, even in the strange bathroom of the family therapist's office. The soap, toweling, and other accoutrements are of considerable interest to the young child. But bathroom and toilet functions may not be regarded as acceptable play by adults. Such necessary activities and interests of young children may become additional fodder for exclusionary therapeutic practices.

Reading about play may be of some assistance in overcoming reluctance to include children in family therapy. The next chapter will search the family therapy literature for play and children in family therapy. This literature is not extensive. We will discuss the sparse, explicit references, and search for hidden references pertaining to young children in family therapy.

CHAPTER NOTE

1) It is not a mistake or an unformed or accidental omission that this example is described in a "father-son" relationship. In my experience, mothers are not usually encouraged to increase their sports or other play activities with sons. Such references are not usually found either in verbal descriptions of therapeutic practice or in the literature.

3

In Search of Children and Play: Through the Family Therapy Literature

> . . . said the (Red) Queen, "Now, here, you see, all the running you can do, to keep in the same place. If you want to get somewhere else, you must run at least twice as fast as that!"
>
> –Carroll (1871) 1941, p. 41

Readers may recall the Red Queen in *Alice in Wonderland*, who had to run very fast just to stay in the same place. In this chapter, we will run as fast as we can, if not twice as fast, since a normal everyday pace through the rapidly increasing family therapy literature will not get us "somewhere else," and we do want to get there – specifically, to young children and play. Sometimes the family therapy literature acts in accord with the Red Queen's descriptions in the reviews and summaries of the literature: They run as fast as they can and end up in the same place! This chapter will also run in place, but only long enough for a good warm-up, since warm-ups are so important for playing a good game!

In this chapter, first we will warm up with a general overview and then narrow the focus to a search for some of the sprinkled references to children and play amongst the larger body of family therapy publications. The overview will include some of the books and articles that have become "classics" in family therapy. Classics are books or articles that in my opinion and by fairly general consensus, over the relatively short history of the family therapy field, have been deemed worthy or important enough to be "musts" for those who wish to be informed about family therapy. Then we will get more intensively acquainted with the very few articles that are specifically about children, play, and family therapy.

But first, a disclaimer, which is particularly directed toward those readers who already "know" the literature. We recognize that to know the literature and to cover even the classics is very difficult, if not impossible, without making some arbitrary choices. The acquaintanceship that follows is selective and certainly not all-inclusive. The principle of selection is this author's judgment that these writings will help further an understanding of young children in family therapy, which is, after all, the main purpose of this volume.

THE PIONEERS AND THE CLASSICS

> *It is not the function of the pioneer to say the last word, but to say the first word.*
>
> -Guntrip, 1971, p. 3

The family therapy field as such had its birth as a distinct clinical area of interest, therapeutic practice, and research in the mid-1950s (Note 1). The pioneer family therapists were brave in breaking previously inflexible psychotherapeutic practices about who should be treated and how. The pioneers progressed rapidly from initial research endeavors that were based on simultaneous therapeutic involvement with mother and child, to involvement of the entire family. Some of their writings have become family therapy classics or landmark publications. One of the earliest landmarks, Ackerman's *The Psychodynamics of Family Life*, was published in 1958. Other early publications include: Bell's monograph, *Family Group Therapy* (1961) and the classic text, *Conjoint Family Therapy* by Satir, which was published shortly thereafter in 1964.

An earlier interesting and somewhat neglected article, entitled "The Study and Reduction of Group Tension in the Family," was published in 1949 (Bowlby, 1949). It was published in a social science journal, *Human Relations*, rather than a family therapy publication, but its inclusion in Erickson and Hogan's *Family Therapy: An Introduction to Theory and Techniques* (1976), a collection of reprinted major articles, indicates that it was noticed as a significant pioneer theoretical contribution.

There were faily well-defined working groups connected with equally important pioneers on the East and West coasts, with a few scattered in between and in other places. The West Coast group, which included Bateson, Jackson, Haley, and Satir, among others, started their family therapy endeavors in an in-patient hospital with the "family" consisting of mother and child, an older hospitalized adolescent. On the East Coast, Ackerman and others included young children in their whole family therapy treatment from the outset.

There are two historical overview articles that organize and describe the early pioneer years and the subsequent growth of the field: Guerin's "Family Therapy: The First Twenty-five Years" (Guerin, 1976); and "Historical Perspectives" (Erickson & Hogan, 1976). A third, more recent informative survey, "The History of Professional Marriage and Family Therapy," appears in Gurman and Kniskern's *The Handbook of Family Therapy* (1981). Sager and Kaplan's (eds.) *Progress in Group and Family Therapy* (1972) is another volume in which the family therapy portion is a good partial survey.

After a few years, distinct schools, branches, or brands of family therapy began to emerge. At present, there is considerable variety and some confusion within the field. The acknowledged mixtures, if they are such, are often called "eclectic," as they combine different ingredients from the strategic, structural, contextually-based, communication-oriented, behaviorally-derived, and other brands of therapy. As I said earlier, only certain aspects of a few of these have been included in this chapter as they contribute to our understanding of young children in family therapy.

Nathan Ackerman—(East Coast branch)

> *A strange paradox marks the question of the participation of children in the family therapeutic interview . . . without engaging the children in a meaningful interchange across the generations, there can be no family therapy.*
>
> -Ackerman, 1970, p. 407

Ackerman has been designated the "Father of family therapy," and I agree! His work with families began before the inception and subsequent development of the family therapy field. In 1938, he published a paper, "The Unity of the Family." Both of his books, *The Psychodynamics of Family Life* (1958) and *Treating the Troubled Family* (1966), are classics. In Ackerman's books and his many other publications, children are always considered a vital part of family life and treatment. This was additionally emphasized in the process of home visits that he included as a method of studying the entire family. In 1958, in a statement of basic philosophy that deserves our current attention, Ackerman declared:

27

None of us lives alone. Those who try are foredoomed; they disintegrate as human beings . . . life is . . . a shared and sharing experience. In the early years this sharing occurs exclusively with members of your family. The family is the basic unit of growth and experience, fulfillment or failure. It is also the basic unit of illness and health. . . . " (p. 1) (Note 2)

Ackerman and others in the East Coast branch have continued to be a potent influence on the family therapy field. The Ackerman Institute has always included young children in their family therapy sessions and in their training. A recent example of this influence will be found in the discussion of a paper by Donald Bloch, presently Director of the Ackerman Institute, in the section on specific references (see *Our Search Rewarded*, pp. 42-43).

Virginia Satir—(West Coast branch)

Family therapists deal with family pain.

-Satir, 1967, p. 1

Virginia Satir is often designated the "Mother of family therapy" and I agree! It is fortunate that both so-called family therapy "parents" included young children in their early family therapy endeavors. However, as we have stated previously, our intent is not to create another family of family therapists, or to otherwise classify the leaders in the field, but to sample the family therapy literature with a particular orientation, the known family therapists who do include younger children and play in their family therapy practice and writings, and to discuss some others by contrast (Note 3).

Satir's classic volume, *Conjoint Family Therapy*, was originally published in 1964 and last revised in 1983. In this early and seminal volume, the chapter entitled "Including the Children in Family Therapy" is particularly noteworthy. This chapter discusses the first interview including children in considerable detail. The book's theoretical orientation places an emphasis on disturbances of communication patterns within families and the family's disentanglement and change in the process of treatment. Satir's therapeutic technique and practice emphasize verbal techniques. Play, as such, is not specifically mentioned, although children of all ages are included in her therapeutic sessions. In the revised edition, Satir mentions in her last chapter "Dancing, body movement, exercises, drama and games" as important therapeutic experiences, which could be considered play experiences for whole families if used in that way.

Bateson, Jackson, Weakland, Haley, Satir—
(West Coast/Palo Alto branch)

> *To describe families, the most appropriate analogy would seem to be the self-corrective system governed by family members influencing each other's behavior and thereby establishing rules and prohibitions for that particular family system. Such a system tends to be error-activated.*
>
> > –Haley, 1957, p. 73

An important, well-known, and early branch of the developing family therapy field, which started in the early 1950s in Palo Alto, included Bateson, Jackson, Haley, Weakland, Satir, and others. This West Coast group, with the leading influence of Bateson (1961), developed a particularly strong and important theoretical orientation derived from general systems theory (Miller, 1969; von Bertalanffy, 1968). Some basic systems concepts, e.g., that each of the interacting elements of a system systematically affects all parts of the system and that the whole is more than the sum of its elements, became generally accepted (Phillips, 1980).

In the ensuing years, general systems theory and, more specifically, the principal concepts of family systems theory have become the theoretical base for the entire field of family therapy (Note 4). Controversy and argument continue in family therapy circles about the place of other theories, such as psychodynamically-oriented or behavior theories, with much fervor and partisan energy. However, two basic concepts of family systems theory, which were explicated in those early years, have continued to be important conceptual cornerstones in family therapy of all kinds: 1) family homeostasis, and 2) double-bind communication. Since the following basic, landmark definitions from early articles have not been substantially modified, they deserve attention in their original form:

1) Family homeostasis.

> *The term* family homeostasis *is chosen from the concept of Claude Bernard, and Cannon because it implies the* relative constancy of the internal environment, *a constancy, however, which is maintained by the continuous interplay of dynamic forces.*
>
> > –Jackson, 1957, p. 5 (author's emphasis)

29

The concept of family homeostasis extended a homeostatic mechanism from biology and physiology to the family as a unit. Family interaction, particularly communication, is viewed (in family systems theory) as a closed information system in which variations in input and behavior are fed back in order to correct the response of the system, the family unit.

Family homeostasis implies a series of alterations in family functions, initially set off by a major internal or external change, resulting in a return to a *previous* form of stability. This is an "error-activated" model in which, after an "input," the system adjusts and returns to a previously set level (*see* Haley, 1957 as quoted above). The concept of family homeostasis is useful in understanding the consistency and stability of family patterns in the face of external or internal stress. However, when the concept of family development is added to our understanding of families, family homeostasis becomes insufficient as an overall concept. Family development implies a series of progressive levels to which a system has to progressively adjust rather than remain at one level. Thus, the family homeostasis patterns may remain constant within levels of family development but not between successive stages (Zilbach, 1979).

2) Double-bind communication.

A double-bind message, the simultaneous transmission of contradictory messages, is a family communication pattern that has received considerable attention in both the family therapy and the research literature. This concept was originally described in families with a schizophrenic member (Bateson et al., 1956). Double-bind communication is of more general interest, however, as a mechanism of family interchange and a focus of therapeutic intervention. The term double-bind is now often used loosely for simple contradictory statements, and has entered everyday parlance as an action: "to double-bind someone."

The original definition clarifies and specifies the more complex meaning of double-bind communication:

1) When the individual is involved in an intense relationship; that is, a relationship in which he feels it is vitally important that he discriminate accurately, what sort of message is being communicated so that he may respond appropriately.

2) And, the individual is caught in a situation in which the other person in the relationship *is expressing two orders of message and one of these denies the other.*

3) And, the individual is *unable to comment* on the messages

being expressed to correct his discrimination of what order of message to respond to, i.e., he cannot make a meta-communicative statement. (Weakland, 1960; author's emphasis)

Notice that this definition includes and requires that not only must all characteristics be present, *but also that the family member in the double-bind respond.* Although this pattern has been deemed universally important in families, double-bind messages toward or from younger children have not been studied (Mishler & Waxler, 1968).

There is no doubt that children are considered, in general, as a part of the family system. But the early history of this West Coast/Palo Alto branch of family therapy specifically consisted of working with a subsystem of parents and "child" – a late adolescent or young adult schizophrenic. Thus, this brand of rapidly developing, systems-oriented family work did not include young children. A systems orientation often seems to imply the idea, paraphrased perhaps simplistically, that since a system is all-inclusive, children will be helped when we treat the adult or parental parts of the system. To paraphrase one family therapist who, when asked to explain the exclusion of young children, stated, "All parts of the system are changed when any part is modified" (Fulweiler, 1967, p. 20). In this major branch or school of family therapy, young children were and often continue to be excluded with a theoretical justification for this therapeutic practice.

Since our concern in this volume is with explicit *inclusion* of young children in family therapy, we will now discuss the schools or branches of family therapy that *do* include young children and play as essential parts of the treatment process.

Salvador Minuchin and his Colleagues

> Only the family, society's smallest unit, can change and yet maintain enough continuity to rear children who will not be "strangers in a strange land," who will be rooted firmly enough to grow and to adapt.
>
> –Minuchin, 1974, p. 47

A pioneer in family treatment, Minuchin and his colleagues have always included children as part of the "structure" of the whole family. Their work has led to the development of an important school or brand of family therapy that is now called "structural family therapy," which by its very nature includes children. An initial definition of structural family therapy is listed as follows:

31

"Structural family therapy" is directed toward changing the organization of the family. When the structure of the family group is transformed, the position of members in that group are altered accordingly. As a result, each individual experience is changed. (Minuchin, 1974, p. 2)

The question of the appropriate age for inclusion of children does not arise since the structure of the entire family is the unit of Minuchin's treatment. Structural family theory emphasizes the importance of particular configurations or structures within families, which are called "subsystems." The "executive subsystem" usually consists of the parents; the children create a "sibling subsystem." The sibling subsystem serves as the first arena for experimenting with peer relationships and includes the functions of support, negotiation, cooperation, competition, and the recognition of skills on the one hand and isolating and scapegoating on the other (Minuchin, 1974).

For our purposes, Minuchin takes particular notice of young children and emphasizes the transactions of security, nurturance, and guidance for the young children within the family, in contrast to the older children who are in the world outside the family making contacts and contracts. Structural family therapy is the only branch of family therapy to take particular theoretical note of young children in the sibling subsystem with a special place, a "further division" for the younger children (Minuchin, 1974).

Structural family therapists have explicit permission, if not encouragement, to play as well as to talk. Since play is not often described in the literature, the following clinical vignette from a structural family therapy session is noteworthy:

In a family . . . the spouses continually attack each other in escalating conflicts, which plateau only when the parents unite with one of their adolescent children. The therapist was able to deflect this dysfunctional pattern *by having the parents bring in only the three children under six*. For three sessions, therapists, parents, and children sat on the floor [playing] building towers and racing cars. Among the youngsters, it was possible to introduce a sense of support between the parents that was impossible with the previous grouping. (Minuchin, 1974, p. 134; author's emphasis)

The crucial functions of including the young children are clearly evident. In this unusual example, we note that the older verbal adolescent children were *excluded* from these few important play sessions, not the younger children as is much more usual. The use of the young children to build support

32

between the parents is an example of young children as allies and co-therapists, which will be discussed further in the next chapter. The children's play is the therapeutic means for building support not only with the children but "between" the parents.

Minuchin explicitly invites all members of the household, including the youngest, to the first family session. He mentions the use of play materials, small chairs and quiet toys, and also the importance of specifically noticing the youngest children in the initial family interview. He instructs the therapist to notice each family member, even though the youngest may not be asked to verbally present a view of the family problems. Also emphasized is the need to make the youngest, i.e., the very young child, feel included, perhaps by gesture rather than words in the initial family sessions (Minuchin, 1974, p. 209). This is discussed more extensively in Chapter 7 in the section entitled, "Hello".

Bits and pieces of play are occasionally included within other structural case descriptions of families. However, they are difficult to find, incomplete, and not marked by any special attention. In one of the previously mentioned volumes (Guerin, 1976), Minuchin, in structural action, is described by Hoffman in a brief example of play with hand puppets. Minuchin directs the mother to get down on the floor and play with her misbehaving daughter. She does, but soon begins to criticize. Minuchin then invites the father to play in a structural rearrangement of this play sequence. The therapist comments on the father's gentle play with his daughter, who is behaving "like an angel" (Hoffman, in Guerin 1976, p. 514). Minuchin's inclusion of the young child and his use of the play are noteworthy. Without the child, the therapist would not have been able to observe and utilize Mother's criticism and Father's gentle play. (Further discussion of play and young children in Montalvo and Haley's paper, "In Defense of Child Therapy," is included in the last Section of this chapter.)

Carl Whitaker

> There is something about getting down on the floor with a five-year-old that does things to the delusion of grandeur with which adult patients ensnare [family therapists]. Children tend to break up the compulsive devotion to words, to increase [their] personal participation through the use of toys as objective symbols and by body contact. . . . It's easy to be personal and loving with a five-year-old and the satisfactions tempt one back into the conviction that people are worth knowing.
>
> –Whitaker, 1981, p. 206

Carl Whitaker is an openly playful therapist, and, in addition, he is explicit and particularly emphatic about the importance he attributes to play. He states that a "family must learn how to play . . . and that the function of play is not as a leftover for spare time but that play must be present to maintain health and facilitate growth" (Whitaker, 1981, p. 200).

He repeatedly expresses not only enthusiasm about young children, but also a preference for being with younger ones under five or six years of age. He describes playing, for example, in a session with a four-year-old, as a powerful experience that may be important to other family members and as a standard therapeutic intervention in his brand of family therapy (Whitaker, in Gurman & Kniskern, 1967, pp. 309–310).

The kind of play Carl Whitaker enjoys may not, however, be fun for all family therapists! But, clearly, it is very enjoyable for Whitaker and his cotherapists, and only his own words can capture these therapeutic play sessions:

> I started playing with a boy, and I didn't mind his hitting me and tearing the pipe out of my mouth and that sort of thing. Everytime I'd light up my lighter, he'd spit on it, until I had a handful of spit, and Mother was sitting over there in her compulsive way, just having fits. . . . (1967, p. 335)

I will quote Whitaker in some detail because he is such an enthusiast and one of our few strong allies in regard to children and play. The following descriptions are unusual, not only in their extensive inclusion of younger children, but also in the many details of play. Even the structure of the room is explicitly organized for one of his particular kinds of play: physical "play-battling":

> We preserve playing space in the middle of the family room for children or for adults since the process usually involves physical interactions, i.e., arm wrestling, seating changes, or play therapy on the floor. (1981, p. 207)

Whitaker and his colleagues, but especially Whitaker himself, have developed a fondness for this special kind of play, which he named "play-battling":

> We have almost developed a technique for working with omnipotent children in family therapy. It involves overpowering the children and turning them back into little kids again. . . . Their sense of omnipotence is extended to include the therapist. They begin

to challenge us and, at that point, we start anticipating a fight. The fight may start as a tease, then gradually becomes more real. While we start off strategically, the confrontation has never stayed technical for either one of us. Tussling with the children might be compared to a handball game. No matter how many times we play, the excitement that it sparks is always real. . . . (Keith & Whitaker, 1977, p. 120)

A lot of play-battling focuses on Whitaker. Details of his play technique include:

We do not let kids win. If they bite, we bite back or push their arms into their mouths. We talk silly and expand their sadistic fantasies of tearing heads off, poking eyes, or knocking brains out. . . . (Keith & Whitaker, 1977, p. 120)

Other kinds of play follow play-battling in his family therapy sessions:

. . . Later on it got so that they [the children] were not really afraid of the fight. In fact, they would use it as a way to relax in the beginning of an interview. As the physical fighting began to quiet down, they started into fantasy play with each other and alone. They drew pictures and brought dreams to the therapy hours. This play therapy with the children occupied much of the first four months of [family] therapy. (Keith & Whitaker, 1977, p. 121)

These and other descriptions of play by Carl Whitaker include both young and somewhat older children. The progression from play-battling to pictures and dreams is worthy of note. Unfortunately, Whitaker does not describe the pictures or report the dreams. However, pictures will be seen in this volume in Chapters 5 and 6.

The reaction of Whitaker's co-therapist, Augustus Napier, to such play-battles, stating that he felt "tremendous relief" just sitting and watching Whitaker play, is heartening (Napier, 1977, p. 136). Napier's comments on sitting and watching are of interest. Each therapist who works with young children in family therapy develops comfort and skill with slightly different play techniques. Observation of other therapists may ease discomfort with play, as Napier's comments indicate. Whitaker is the only proponent of play-battling in the literature, although other therapists have indicated their pleasure with play (Ackerman, 1970; Bergel, Gass, & Zilbach, 1968; Bloch, 1976).

CASEBOOKS OF FAMILY THERAPY

In the course of this brief journey through the literature in our search for children and play, we take particular note of two casebooks of family therapy: 1) *Techniques of Family Therapy* (Haley & Hoffman, 1967); and, 10 years later, 2) *Family Therapy: Full-Length Case Studies* (Papp, 1977). These books, although not specifically addressed to our topic, include valuable descriptions and transcripts of actual family interviews and commentary by therapists which do contain some references to or descriptions of children and play.

Techniques of Family Therapy

The format of *Techniques of Family Therapy* (Haley & Hoffman, 1967) is a transcript of an initial family therapy interview and interviews with Fulweiler, Satir, Jackson, Whitaker, and the team of Pitman, Flomenhaft, and DeYoung. This book is useful for our purposes because there are a few young children among the mixed-age cases. In addition, the therapists were specifically asked about including "whole" families with children.

In the first chapter, Charles Fulweiler takes a clear position on *not* working with whole families:

> . . . When a child is the problem, I have found it more productive to treat the child with his parents as a triad, rather than bring all the other siblings in, though I like to see the others at least once. That's why, in this family, *I didn't include the younger girl in treatment.* I've worked through several families by taking each child in a threesome with the parents *as he gets old enough to participate.* (Haley & Hoffman, 1967, p. 20; author's emphasis)

Fulweiler does not give any explicit criteria to determine what age a child has to attain to be "old enough to participate." He does include the small children for one interview in order to observe how the parents "handle" their children. His emphasis is clearly on parents and on working with "their own problems." Young children are not included by Fulweiler until they are "old enough." While Fulweiler does not specify the characteristics of "old enough," they are likely to be sit-in-a-chair-then-talk, adult characteristics.

Fulweiler explains further and invokes the principle of "family homeostasis" discussed earlier (see pp. 29–30) as an explanation of this therapeutic practice:

I would never see a family of more than three all through therapy. The number of interactions is too great. . . . Well, if you accept the idea of family homeostasis, of a family system, it doesn't matter which section of it you're dealing with. If you change the interpersonal balance of one triad, you will effect the whole system. (Haley & Hoffman, 1967, p. 20)

I have quoted Fulweiler in some detail to give a clear example of a family therapist's use of family systems theory to explain his exclusion of young children. It is particularly important to note his comment about observing a young couple "handling" their children. But what about the young child's reaction to parental "handling"? Does each young child's reactions to being "handled" also affect the family system? The child's reactions and feelings are as important and have as much right in family therapy as the actions and reactions of the "handling" parental couple.

In addition, Fulweiler comments that the number of interactions are too great for the therapist! But family life is inevitably complex and made up of a great "number of interactions" with which family members live and encounter daily as these complications multiply. No doubt there is an effect on the triad and beyond the triad to all other members of the family. But, in this instance, those other actions go unobserved by the family therapist who, as a result, also does not have to be concerned with them. A child who becomes quiet and compliant with a new type of "handling" may not be making much noise but may be in psychological trouble.

A contrasting approach is found in the next chapter of this first family casebook. The therapist in this whole family case is Virginia Satir who includes children with no lower age limitation:

Interviewer: Did the children come to the first session?
Mrs. S: Yes . . . there was Gail, 22; Gary [17], the labeled patient; Lois, 12; and Tim, five. They were nice kids, but pale in spirit, as if they weren't sure what they could or couldn't do. . . . (Hoffman & Haley, 1967, p. 98)

Beyond the initial interview, the interviewer explores Satir's approach to including the whole family:

Interviewer: Did you continue to see the family as a unit through treatment?
Mrs. S: Yes. To understand the meaning of a symptom, I have to see how it fits into the family system.

Interviewer: If the child with the symptom gets better, do you leave him out of treatment and concentrate on the parent?

Mrs. S: No, I don't. I have ambitious goals for therapy. I don't want simply to repair the family. I want to focus on prevention and also to accomplish an expansion of possibilities for each person. (Haley & Hoffman, 1967, p. 98)

This approach is consonant with the philosophy in this book. In particular, Satir mentions prevention and the expansion of the possibilities for each person as a goal for family therapy – and she certainly includes the youngest, the five-year-old child.

In the same family casebook, in the chapter "The Eternal Triangle," Don Jackson holds a contrasting discussion about involving the whole family, although there are no young children in the particular family. As was frequently the case in the early work of the Palo Alto family therapy branch, the family treatment unit consisted of parents and an older adolescent child. The treatment unit in the initial session was the patient, a hospitalized, schizophrenic 18-year-old, and the parents. The other three siblings, ages 17, 15, and 13, were not included in the family treatment. Subsequently, Jackson treated the youngest daughter in individual therapy and then the oldest boy. Dr. Jackson comments:

. . . I felt like a paperhanger with bad glue, running around, never organized the way I would have liked to be.

Interviewer: Do you think you could have avoided this if you had seen them all together from the start?

Dr. J: I don't know. It was an unusual circumstance. All these children were growing up and getting to the point of leaving home. If you see the whole family as a unit, there may be some benefits, but it gets the kids reinvolved. . . . (Haley & Hoffman, 1967, p. 180)

In this instance, the exclusion of the other children is based on a different conception of family development. As Jackson says, the children were getting to the point of "leaving home" and presumably leaving the family. Thus, seeing them together, and getting "reinvolved," is not necessarily beneficial. In my conceptualization of family development this family was in a middle family stage where, as the children are leaving home, they are not leaving the whole family. Once a member of a family always a member of a family but with different characteristics and different functions at different stages of family development (see pp. 6-8 and Zilbach, 1979).

Carl Whitaker is the therapist in Chapter 4. His contrasting orientation and pleasure at the inclusion of young children, which have been extensively discussed earlier in this chapter, again emerge quickly and clearly in this case example that includes several young children:

> . . . I'll be glad to see you and your wife and your son and *your four other kids too*. He [Father] said, "You mean expose those little children to this horrible mess." I said, "Look, they've been living it for years." So we made an appointment for the whole family. . . . (Haley & Hoffman, 1967, p. 267; author's emphasis)

Whitaker emphasizes his position on including the entire family with the "little ones" in his account of his discussion with Mother when she called and questioned him. She thought it was "criminal to bring the little children in." Whitaker states his position unequivocally by asking if she wants to cancel the appointment (Haley & Hoffman, 1967, p. 267)!

The seriousness and importance of play is emphasized in the interviewer's last question and comments to Whitaker:

> Interviewer: Before we end, there is one thing I'd like to bring up. There seems to be a major theme throughout this interview, and that is a quality of playfulness. You seem to be teaching the family how to play: with names, with words, with issues, with each other. You use your relationship with the children as a way of instructing the family how to enjoy themselves.
> Dr. W: That's right. . . . (Haley & Hoffman, 1967, p. 360)

After this emphatic comment, perhaps disbelieving, or unable to get beyond the prevalent opinions about play which have been discussed previously in this book, the interviewer restates Whitaker's position and receives a final strong affirmation about the importance of play:

> Interviewer: . . . but there is another thing about this playing. It is done in a context in which people are in an absolute misery and paying money to get out of it. Yet within that context, you play.

Dr. W: That's true, and that's one of the things people can misunderstand. Sometimes people will say to me, "You don't seem to be taking this seriously," or "Were you kidding when you said that?" I tell them, "This is a life or death job. There is nothing I do here that's for fun. I am dead serious from the time you get here to the time you leave." (Haley & Hoffman, 1967, p. 360)

Thus, our search has been partly rewarded in this casebook of family therapy where some examples of family therapy work that include young children have been found. They are not regarded by the authors or editors of the volumes as being particularly important, but we have described them in some detail to lift them from obscurity for the purpose of including young children in family therapy.

Family Therapy: Full-Length Case Studies

The second landmark casebook, *Family Therapy: Full-Length Case Studies* (Papp, 1977), includes 11 full-length family cases that contain a few young children. In one chapter, "An Identified Patient," Beels mentions an 11-month-old who came to all interviews. However, the description of this very young child, Fiona, and play are minimal:

She stumbled charmingly around my office. . . . (p. 36)
. . . I found it easy to spend a little time playing with Fiona and chatting [with the parents] about things I was interested in. . . . (Papp, 1977, p. 39)

Beels does not give us any further details about play or Fiona; whether or not Jesse and Mary, the parents, also play or how Beels played. It is possible, that in his therapy sessions, Beels was actually teaching them to play, a most important aspect of family life and an explicit goal of family treatment for Whitaker and others. It is clear, however, that Beels not only includes young children, but is comfortable playing with them.

Two important chapters in this casebook contain young children: "The Divorce Labyrinth," and "The Follow-up to the 'Divorce Labyrinth.'" These chapters have been extensively discussed in the previous section on Carl Whitaker. The other families in this casebook contain some youngish children (age eight) but mostly older ones (12-17), and only verbal interactions are described.

OUR SEARCH REWARDED

So far we have emphasized the paucity of articles in the family therapy literature that deal exclusively with young children and/or play in family therapy. However, there are four major articles that explicitly call attention to and discuss young children in family therapy, which I will now review in some detail.

In the first article, "Child Participation in Family Therapy" (1970), Ackerman took a strong position:

> The central importance of the question is self-evident; without engaging the children in a meaningful interchange across the generations, there can be no family therapy . . . in the daily practice of this form of treatment, difficulties in mobilizing the participation of children are a common experience. It is all the more surprising to realize, therefore, . . . that *there is not a single publication devoted to this special theme*. (Ackerman, 1970, p. 407; author's emphasis)

In connection with the attitudes of family therapists toward children, Ackerman discusses the now classic "Hillcrest Family Series" film. Four family therapists, Ackerman, Bowen, Jackson, and Whitaker, were filmed interviewing the same family over a two-day period, each therapist not knowing about the other interviews (Note 5).

Fortunately for our concerns with young children, the children in this film were ages 10, eight, five, and one and a half. Ackerman reports that 20 professionals viewing these interviews thought that two of the therapists did not relate to the children, a third therapist interviewed them minimally, and only one of the four (left unnamed!) "showed strong rapport and actively engaged them (the children) in the treatment of the family as family." Ackerman mentions the known predilection of therapists to have an "age preference" in their therapeutic endeavors. This issue has been discussed in Chapter 1 and is, I believe, more accurately referred to as an age *exclusion* than an age preference.

Ackerman does not discuss play in this article, although he mentions some of the aspects of making contact and introductions with children (see Chapter 7). He concludes on a note of considerable import:

> The mobilization of *effective* participation of child members is essential to the elucidation, stage by stage, of the family war, the alignment and splits in the family group, the hidden conflict of the

parents, the scapegoating, etc. . . . . If they feel protected here and fairly dealt with, their sense of personal importance is gratifying. . . .

Fundamentally, the child's drive for self-expression is a constructive and healing influence for the parents as well. It opens a path for a new way of relating, not only between parents and children, but also between the parents. What is involved is a movement toward a deeper and more appropriate kind of emotional honesty among the [family] members. (Ackerman, 1970, p. 410; author's emphasis)

Notice that Ackerman is commenting on the child's healing effect on the parents. This is most unusual! Our adult-oriented therapeutic culture often totally ignores or does not recognize sufficiently the positive healing effects of children on their parents. Such effects are usually thought of primarily in terms of parental effects on children, both good and bad!

In the second article, "Including the Children in Family Therapy" (1976), Bloch discusses similar issues: the important place of minor (young) children in family therapy, the resistance to inclusion, and the special modes of relating that are needed for younger children. He emphasizes the child's gift for metaphor and vivid expressiveness in an example in which a child, in answer to his question, "How is your life?," says, "like eating out of a broken apple . . . a bad apple" (p. 177). Bloch's examples are delightfully replete with young children, including a poignant example, and a rarity in this literature, of a two-week-old named Adorée.

Bloch also explicitly addresses the use of himself in a playful way. He states that his play will activate emotional, meaningful configurations in the family session. The therapist's explicit use of the "self" is currently a major topic in the psychoanalytic individually-oriented literature. The use of self as an individual therapist has been addressed in regard to parenting, holding, other nurturing activities, and limit setting (Kohut, 1971, 1977; Winnicott, 1958). In family therapy, the use of self is examined only in discussions of the therapist's place, within the family system or outside, and separated by an imposed boundary.

But the playful use of the self by therapist is different in Bloch's example and deserves special attention. Playing with words, joking, and laughing are more familiar than his attention to the larger playful use of the "body-self," which is exemplified by a game of "footsie." Playing with young children may include hands, feet or whole body. There are many children's games like "footsie" and we take special note of Bloch's description because few are reported in the literature. (Some possible origins of the therapist's difficulties with being playful, including games and other forms of play have been discussed on pp. 20–22.)

The third article by Montalvo and Haley, "In Defense of Child Therapy" (1973), particularly discusses the problem of exclusion:

> A child therapy orientation may prevent one of the most recent and common errors of family therapy – that of overfocusing on the couple and losing the child in the process. (p. 234)

The authors state that the marital couple may change but the child may *fail* to change. Moreover, child change is often assumed to be automatic if the marital couple changes. Montalvo and Haley emphasize that the child's contribution is necessary for full resolution of problems. These therapists are taking a position in opposition to other family systems therapists, such as Fulweiler (1967) who state that a change in the parents will inevitably change the child.

An important part of Montalvo and Haley's paper is an extensive discussion and definition of play:

> . . . Play is one of the most important factors in human life, but in child therapy, "play" is a peculiar and deviant form. By definition, play is something that occurs between voluntary participants and has no purpose except the pleasure of the action. This generally accepted definition of play is clearly not applicable to "play therapy." When play is used as a therapeutic tool, it is given a purpose and so by definition becomes something other than play. . . . [It is] a special communication that has different rules from ordinary life. . . . (pp. 235–236)

The authors emphasize both the freedom and suspension of rules during play that allow for change in behavior:

> . . . the toys in the playroom become devices for trial and error experimentation. They not only become expressions of real family issues that can be resolved (as theory has it) in symbolic form, but more importantly, they can become a vehicle for the therapist's instructions as to how to deal with these family issues in reality. . . . (p. 236)

The authors describe a number of examples in which play and fantasy in the safety and privacy of the playroom mirror the actions of the family and,

43

as the child learns to deal through play with harmful family interventions by coping with them in miniature, change occurs. The interactions between therapist and child, child and parent, and parents and therapist are all influenced by these new ways of coping that are learned in the play therapy. Thus, Montalvo and Haley believe that these play changes affect not only the child, but also the entire family. Note the similarity of the strategy used by these authors with the direction of the approach mentioned by Ackerman.

The fourth article in this discussion of specific references to young children in family therapy, Aponte and Hoffman's "The Open Door: A Structural Approach to a Family With an Anorectic Child" (1973), does not include very young children, but does emphasize the importance of the participation of nonsymptomatic children, as well as the entire family. In the family in this case, the children, ages 10 and 12, and the 14-year-old index patient, were being kept young, closely "bundled in," and "bunched" into the family. Unless younger children, particularly the very young, are flagrantly symptomatic, they are frequently considered dispensable in family sessions. The intricacies and subtleties of the involvement of all members, including the youngest child, the 10-year-old in this instance, are well described. At the very end of the interview, after the therapist declared, "We have only 10 minutes," this child, who was completely silent until this point, declared, "I have something to say." A clear, brief message emerged as this heretofor most important family member described "babysitting" his older sisters and being paid for this job by his father! This family had considerable difficulty with appropriate generational boundaries and roles.

The "strategies" of another brand of family therapy that certainly includes children can be found in an article by Haley, "Strategic Therapy When a Child Is Presented as the Problem" (1973). Haley discusses several categories of strategies based on the principle that there is always an overinvolved adult when a child is presented as the problem. The strategies Haley has devised to undo this structure are categorized as: "1) using the peripheral person . . . ; 2) breaking up the dyad with a task . . . ; [and] 3) entering through the parents" (Haley, 1973, pp. 642-643). The emphasis in this article is on specific "tactics" that will get the entire family to change within a brief period of therapeutic intervention.

Two other articles (Guttman, 1975; Villeneuve, 1979), in general, point to the same major issues: the importance of child participation, exclusion, and the lack of documentation and description of methods for involving children. Villeneuve adds some discussion of the necessity for concrete, action-promoting modes of expression. He mentions the use of psychodramatic techniques, audiovisual techniques (video playback), drawing, puppet play, game play, and "sculpting." The latter, arranging the family in a tableau, makes "live family portraits" and, he states, abstract notions become more concrete for the child. He does not specify age, though his emphasis, in this paper, is on latency-age (elementary-school-age) children.

A recent volume, *Questions and Answers in the Practice of Family Therapy* (Gurman, 1981) takes specific note of children in one "Question and Answer." Chasin, in "Involving Latency and Preschool Children in Family Therapy," describes an "ideal" office layout, which includes play material, some ground rules about safety and limit setting, and engaging the children actively through the use of play. He makes an interesting distinction between two kinds of play, and their use: "Real Play," and "Make Believe Play." Real Play is used to transmit historic information and Make Believe Play uses children's imaginations. He feels that these methods of play can be used with "most family approaches which prevail today, except for those which purposefully avoid the active inclusion of children[!]" (Chasin, in Gurman, 1981, pp. 32–35).

There are some other, briefer references to children in Gurman's book. A discussion of photographs of children and their meanings are included in a chapter on the general use of photographs and family albums in family therapy (Entin, in Gurman, 1981, pp. 421–425). Younger children and secrets are mentioned (Sugarman, in Gurman, 1981, p. 43), and the "child identified patient" is also briefly considered (Pinsof, in Gurman, 1981, p. 195).

In the second volume of *Questions and Answers in the Practice of Family Therapy* (Gurman, 1982), this author poses questions about whether and how to include young children and offers some brief answers (Zilbach, in Gurman, 1982).

A recent article published in French, "La thérapie familiale auprès de jeunes enfants" (Guttman, 1983), contains some interesting case examples of work with younger children.

Finally, another specific chapter on this topic, by the author and her colleagues, "The Role of the Young Child in Family Therapy" (Zilbach, Bergel, & Gass, 1972) has served as the foundation for this book so it will not be discussed further. This book does the job!

One last article that includes young children is a bit outside our topic because its subject is family diagnostic interviews rather than family treatment. However, the approach is consistent with our orientation. Serrano, in "A Child-Centered Family Diagnostic Interview" (1979), notes that the temptation to not include nonverbal young children is present for diagnosticians. He emphasizes the importance and benefits of including the nonverbal children:

"When we include the child with the family, in the initial interview, an additional benefit may accrue. The child may become aware that he has not been previously discussed with the therapists and 'judged' and his individual rights have not been restricted" (Serrano, 1979, p. 625).

In looking for children and play, we have met some of the pioneers and dipped into some of the classics. Finally, we have commented on articles that have been written more directly about our subject. Each of these articles has emphasized, in its own way, the importance of including young children in family therapy. This will be discussed in detail in the next chapter in which the importance is taken up in terms of the "critical functions" of young children in family therapy (Zilbach, 1977) (Notes 6 and 7).

CHAPTER NOTES

1) Every field has ancestors, whether they are legitimized by explicit recognition or not. One ancestor, Freud, used the term "family circumstances" in his famous "Dora" case in 1905. He drew attention to the family of his famous patient by stating:

> It follows from the nature of the facts which form the material of psychoanalysis that we are obliged to pay as much attention in our case history to the purely human and social circumstances of our patients as to the somatic data and the symptoms of the disorder. Above all, our interest will be directed to their *family circumstances* – and not only as will be seen later, for the purpose of inquiring into their heredity. (Freud, 1905, p. 18; author's emphasis)

"Little Hans" has been called the first family therapy case. Little Hans had a childhood horse phobia and was treated by his father who discussed and planned the treatment with Freud. Freud did have a conversation with the boy, but the entire family – mother and younger sibling, Hanna – were not included. The father brought a drawing to the consultation, which was later reproduced in the body of the "Little Hans" publication (Freud, 1909). Another ancestor publication is Flugel's *The Psychoanalytic Study of the Family*, which was published in 1921. I have discussed this more extensively elsewhere (Zilbach, 1968).

2) It is nice to see pioneers as they actually work. The movie *The Enemy in Myself* has excerpts from three family interviews with Nathan Ackerman, which were taken over an 18-month period. The family includes mother, father, and two boys. The film is available from the Ackerman Institute for Family Therapy, 149 East 78 Street, New York, NY 10021.

3) Satir, an early and vigorous member of this branch, has spent more recent years developing the "Human Growth Movement," as the Director of the Esalen Institute of California, a central and leading institution within this movement.

4) In a recent publication, Lynn Hoffman reviews existing family systems theory and also attempts an extension of theory with her own ideas (Hoffman, 1981).

5) The Hillcrest Family Series was produced by Van Flack, Birdwhistell, and Schefflin. The movie is available through the Psychological Cinema Register, Pennsylvania State University, University Park, PA, and is a useful training film.
6) Though not a classic, the recent publication of *The Handbook of Family Therapy* (Gurman, 1981) deserves our particular attention. It is a major step in bringing some order to the rapidly emerging morass of family therapy literature. Children are well covered, as is reflected in the index. Play likewise receives some attention.
7) Knowledgeable readers may ask why the article, "Keith: A Case Study of Structural Family Therapy" (Heard, 1978), has not been included in this last section. At the outset, this article seems relevant since the identified patient is an eight-year-old and there is some recognition of the importance of this child. However, very shortly we learn that both the interview with the individual child and conjoint interview with his parents are omitted:

> Although interviews with Keith were an integral part of the entire process of the therapy, and the case should not be considered a complete case presentation without them, the emphasis of this presentation will be on the unfolding of husband and wife transactions and the movement toward dealing with the marital issues in a case in which the child is originally presented as a symptom. (Heard, 1978, p. 340)

Our interest is again stimulated when we are reminded, after some pages of transcript, that ". . . parents and child have been seen together on a regular basis." But there is no description. So, again, we are frustrated, particularly since, in the discussion of the case, we hear that "the 'kids' (are) weights on a pan scale being shifted here and there to restore structural balance between conflicting parents." And finally, children are ". . . 'complications' I believe, anticipated from two sources, one theoretical, and one practical; 1. Since children (under twelve), are such 'special' communicators, their expressions (behavioral, verbal, or playful) and understanding cannot be used as part of the family treatment process. . . . " So we are disappointed by this article and encouraged to complete the work of this book!

.

4

Critical Functions of Young Children in Family Therapy

Jennifer leaps
around boxes and apple trees
chasing the dog who meets her
with balls dropped at her feet
and her body curved
to Jennifer's warmth on the green quilt of the night.

Jennifer's mind listens to details
weaving in and out of her brain like the tendrils
of flowers and leaves. Whatever
confines the pattern in limits of old frames
she fights in the spirit
of plant-tenders leaping walls
to wipe out pests and plagues and fences forever.

Jennifer jumps up and puts her arms
and legs around things that she loves. . . .

-Snyder, 1979, p. 48

Young children are integral parts of the whole family unit and essential components of family structure, and contribute to family functions, style, myths, and history as evoked in the introductory poem, *Jennifer*. This chapter

49

narrows our focus to the specific critical functions of young children in family therapy. In order to avoid misunderstandings at the outset, this chapter is *not* critical of young children, nor do I intend to criticize the functions of young children in family therapy. Rather, I mean by critical the *crucial* and, at times, decisive and pivotal functions of young children in family therapy. Secondly, by function we mean "the normal or characteristic action of anything," and in this case "anything" is specifically young children. The term "function" gains additional meaning and emphasis in the following definition: "A special duty or performance required of a person or thing in the course of work or activity" (Webster, 1979), which is relevant to young children in the family and in family therapy.

An additional definition of function is also relevant: "A thing that depends on and varies with something else" (Webster, 1979). Thus, the term function includes the characteristic of interdependence, when one quantity depends upon another as is the case in so many aspects of family life. This definition emphasizes the specialness of the duty or performance which is so important in our use of the term "critical functions" of young children. So the term "critical function" seems particularly felicitious as it combines several qualities – crucial, decisive, and interdependence, all important in understanding children in a family, and, in this context, particularly young children in family therapy (Note 1).

CRITICAL FUNCTIONS OF YOUNG CHILDREN IN FAMILY THERAPY: DEFINITIONS AND DESCRIPTIONS

What are the critical functions of young children in family therapy? The following definitions and descriptions represent our current understanding of critical functions of young children.

This list of critical functions has changed over the years. No function has been deleted. However, our growing understanding has expanded both the number and specific characteristics of each function and is likely to continue to expand in future years.

Tip of the Iceberg

Though the tip of the iceberg is small and clearly visible, it is actually only a tiny part of the whole, much larger entity of the iceberg. The main body of the iceberg lies hidden below the surface of the water and is not immediately apparent. A careful watch must be kept for icebergs! When they are detected an immediate report is sent out to all ships that are in adjacent waters.

This image is a good one for families with small children. One of the most important critical functions of young children is that they often provide access to family problems by making the problems very visible to others. One form of "tip of the iceberg" is as "symptom-bearers," which is actually only a small portion of the entirety of family difficulties. The actions and activities of young children are often easily and clearly visible outside of the immediate family to others in day care, nursery school, and other community activities. The family is told to seek help for the child and thus, this small tip, the young child, functions as the critical access to the larger, often more painful problems. School problems and learning difficulties of the young may seem easier to reveal to the extrafamilial world since they may be more acceptable to the family than more serious or complicated neurotic or psychotic adult difficulties.

Though children can be the "tip," prominent spokespeople for family problems, in ways other than being symptom-bearers, clinicians are most familiar with this form of critical function by children. However, after the symptom-bearing function has been eased or diminished in family sessions, nonsymptomatic children will often continue to function in other ways to be the tip for as yet invisible problems (Note 2).

Beyond the Tip of the Iceberg

Just "beyond the tip of the iceberg," below the surface, well disguised in the larger body of the family, serious difficulties may exist which involve other children and/or other older members of the family. The "symptom-bearer," "labelled," or "identified patient" may be the healthiest child – actually a flag bearer of health in the form of symptoms. It is critical to include all the family members in therapy to begin to comprehensively understand and treat family dysfunction. Thus, young children may function in a critical fashion beyond the tip of the iceberg to express serious, unrecognized difficulties. It becomes crucial to include all children in diagnostic sessions in order to properly assess the total family situation:

> In the A family there was a five-year-old-child and a "symptomatic" preadolescent. The well-behaved, "perfect" five-year-old sister of the referred child, a noisy, delinquent preteenager, quietly sat drawing. Although seemingly ignoring the lively conversation in the room, she noticed the therapist watching her artwork. Soon this five-year-old produced a picture of a human figure, not clearly

51

identifiable as either male or female, holding a long whip. When asked about this picture, she concretely and vividly described a whip recently purchased by her parents. They responded to this description by saying, "The whip is a joke – we playfully chase after the children with it."

The picture and ensuing discussion opened a hitherto unrevealed area of serious family problems. This was a family in which there was physical and other abuse of the younger children, in addition to the more apparent delinquent behavior of the preteenager.

Allies and "Co-therapists"

Children function in families as allies and direct explainers and, thus become co-therapists since they can make statements unclouded by adult obfuscation and sophistication. It is important to recognize that these statements about therapeutic alliance may be made most clearly, not only in words, but in play and other forms of expressive activity:

> In the B family, a young, active child made a lot of noise running around the therapy room until he gained the full attention of the therapist and all other family members. Then he stopped and carefully scratched out some numbers on the blackboard over and over again. The chalk made an insistent, grating sound. The therapist noted aloud that the numbers were the date of the next family therapy session. When asked, the child blurted out, "I want to come but my parents aren't coming anymore." The negative feelings and actual specific intention not to continue treatment had not been mentioned by either parent or any other family member.

Some emotions are most difficult to express in words. Feelings of emptiness, loneliness, and the more general experience of not being loved enough, or of general deprivation may be expressed more openly and clearly by young children with the assistance of play materials:

> Paper, pencils, crayons and play-dough were in ample supply in the first session with the C family with several young children. The parents watched, said nothing, and took no action, as the children fought steadily and bitterly over the use and possession of each item. This unending and unchecked behavior, which expressed,

"there is never enough," seemed to represent unspoken needs for love and attention which were shared by all members of the family.

Emptiness is clearly expressed in Photo 4.4 (see p. 59). The lines are very thin, and the spaces in which the sad figure lies all alone remain empty. Concepts of self and representations of important others, e.g., parents and siblings, may be presented more easily by children in pictures than words. Artwork and expression will be discussed with accompanying plates in Chapters 5 and 6.

Children are often expert in being therapeutic alliance builders – even very young babies can do this. A good example of alliance building, discussed earlier, appears in *Family Therapy: Full-Length Case Studies* (Papp, 1977). The therapist, Dr. Beels, played with an 11-month-old throughout the session. This play provided a comfortable demonstration of safety in the grandfather-therapist role which was sorely needed in the early phases of family therapy with this very tense and difficult family. Children enlist alliance in family treatment in many ways. There is another case illustration in the same book (Papp, 1977), also described earlier, of Whitaker having serious fights with two children as an essential part of alliance building in the family therapy.

Young children may be effective as co-therapists by describing and clarifying family mechanisms:

> A young child painted quietly in a corner as the parents' and his teenage sibling's voices escalated in a fight about privileges and rules in the D family. As the voices reached a feverish pitch, the young painter dropped and broke a paint container. The mother turned away from the conversation toward him. Quickly the young child yelled, "See – she's going to get me now and he (the teenager) will get away!" This mechanism had occurred many times in earlier sessions. Now, the young child put an important family mechanism into a few words.

Early Detection

The inclusion of the young children in family therapy may bring troubles that are just developing to the attention of the family therapist. These first stages of problems might otherwise go undetected, and early detection may prevent later, more serious consequences:

A four-year-old, asymptomatic girl in the E family referred for behavior problems of an other older sibling, wanted to get some water from the bathroom to continue her painting. She asked her mother to go with her because she explained, "I am afraid to go alone." The mother, without hesitation, agreed to go with the child, although she was right in the middle of speaking. The therapists intervened and told the girl that it was important for Mother to remain in the room. They suggested that the child try to get the water by herself and assured her that help was available if she needed it. She was able to perform this task on her own and returned to the therapy room visibly pleased.

These actions led directly and naturally to the subject of the child's fears, which were discussed after she returned to the room. She and her parents acknowledged the increasing occurrence of fears which inhibited the child's outdoor play and other actions. When asked how she felt her parents could best help her deal with her fears, the little girl replied that she wanted them to help her get used to the fears.

In the discussion that followed, the mother revealed that she, too, suffered from multiple fears and phobias and often responded to her daughter as if there really were something to fear. The father then mentioned that the maternal grandmother, who had a close relationship with her granddaughter, also reacted to minor difficulties with disproportionate anxiety which often approached panic. Thus, not only did the mother learn how her attitudes perpetuated her daughter's fears, but a family pattern spanning at least three generations was revealed for further therapeutic investigation. The play, which had begun as an expressive activity (painting) and had quickly turned into a defensive maneuver (going out of the room and trying to pull Mother out), became an opportunity for the discussion of an intergenerational family problem and observation of the manner in which it was passed from one generation to the next. In addition, it seemed likely that the child's fears, if undetected, would have become more entrenched over time. She was a likely candidate for a school phobic reaction and/or other more general separation difficulties in her later years.

The recognition of qualities in each family member as part of early detection has an important positive aspect. Certain qualities in individual family members may be enhanced in family sessions and result in an expansion of potential possibilities that otherwise might not have occurred. In other words, early detection may be of assets and potentials rather than problems and symptoms.

The Dynamics and Quality of Whole Family Interactions: Whole Family Understanding

A therapist cannot expect to understand a family's current situation, past history, or future hopes and fears unless s/he knows all members of the family. The entire family as a unit participates in family development. This development is epigenetic: The tasks of the whole family, at each stage of the family life cycle, are different, and build upon each other. Consequently, the way in which the younger, and even the youngest, as well as the older members of the family participate at specific stages of family development will greatly influence family life in subsequent stages. The inclusion of the younger children as an integral part of an entire family is essential to the therapist's understanding of the family's past developmental history and current situation, sense of total family identity, and making help available to all members of the family. (See pp. 6–8 for Family Development: Stages of Family Life Cycle.)

As I said in an earlier chapter, my orientation toward family problems is that there may be an impasse, restriction, or other problem in family development. All family members participate in family development and, indeed, all family members participate in some way in an impasse or difficulties.

Role modeling by the therapist – demonstrating parental behavior in the presence of the entire family – is, at times, a therapist's proper function. But the step prior to modeling is most important, that is, the understanding of whole family interactions. It seems obvious to ask how you would know what to teach if you don't know what you think is wrong or missing. And yet it seems that many times that is what happens in family work with incomplete families, i.e., without the presence of young children.

Understanding Whole Family Interactions

Inclusion of all family members, and specifically all of the younger children, helps therapists understand *whole family interactions*. The inclusion of all children, especially the younger and asymptomatic children, often leads one of the children to elucidate the dynamics of current whole family functioning or dysfunctioning. Sometimes the message is dramatic:

A nonreferred six-year-old girl in the F family made a face in response to mild teasing by her father. When the therapist asked her about this teasing she said, "Ya, my father teases me. Then I get my younger brother, and he has a tantrum and a fight with my mother, and then my mother and father fight about him." With that statement she elucidated an important recurrent pattern in the family's daily life. She added "We all do that all the time." The referral problem had been limited to the behavior problems of her younger brother.

The previous example is an illustration of how children are capable of serious and well-thought-out opinions about their families, and of understanding and then describing complex family mechanisms.

The following photographs will illustrate pictorially the critical functions of young children in family therapy.

CRITICAL FUNCTIONS

I. Tip of the Iceberg

The oldest child, referred for "behavior problems," is making a disgusted face while drawing as the parents describe her troublesome, obstinate behavior. The father's hand motion accompanies a discouraged statement, "I don't know what we can do about her." The other children quietly busy themselves. (Photo 4.1)

In this picture, this "problem" child has picked up a gun in order to shoot the "parent" dolls in the dollhouse. The youngest sister, on the couch, shows displeasure at this direct display of hostility toward the parents. (Photo 4.2)

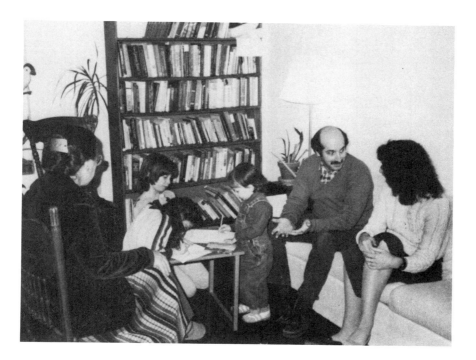

Photo 4.1

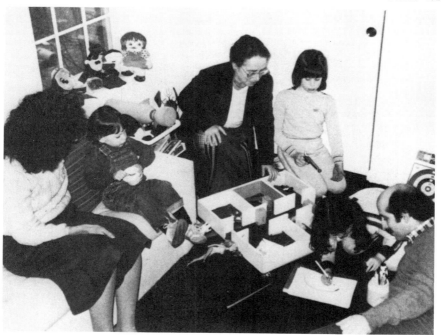

Photo 4.2

57

II. Beyond the Tip

The "problem" child is pointing to the "other trouble" – her "normal" baby sibling, who exchanges startled glances with her sister. The third sibling looks toward the therapist. (Photo 4.3)

In this picture as the eldest's pointing finger becomes more insistent and accusing, the baby draws back against Mother and looks down to avoid the oldest sister's accusations. The baby had serious eating and sleeping difficulties which had not been regarded as problematic by the parents. They were first "pointed" out in a description by the "problem" child. (Photo 4.4)

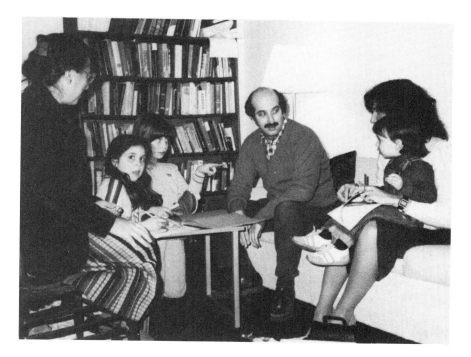

Photo 4.3

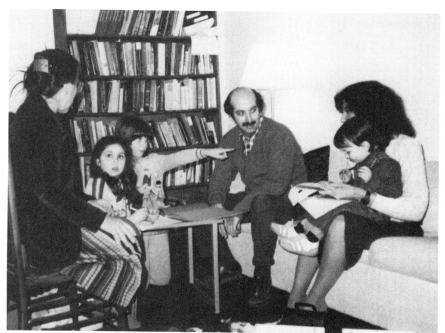

Photo 4.4

III. Allies and "Co-therapists"

The "problem" child is telling a puppet story with Father in which, with a smile, she describes their family interaction through the puppet play. (Photo 4.5)

In this picture, she explains directly to the therapist how Father accuses her of misdoings when Mother "feels bad." Mother has bouts of depression in which she becomes nonfunctional and bedridden. (Photo 4.6)

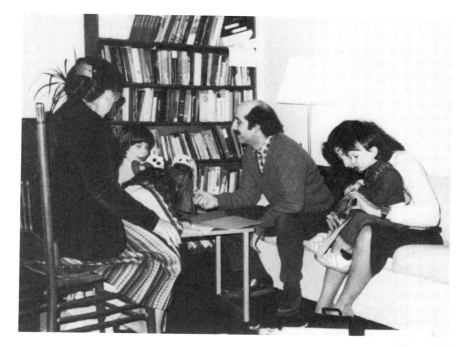

Photo 4.5

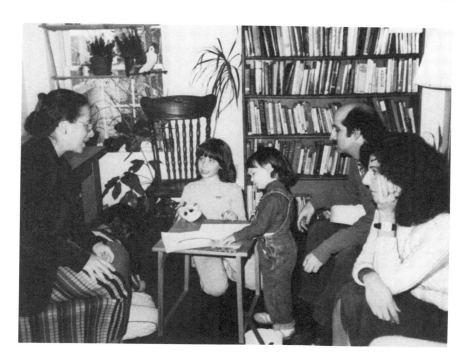

Photo 4.6

61

IV. Early Detection

The baby leaves the scene of action, takes her toys onto the floor, and turns away from potential comforters. Attempts to bring her back produce tears and tantrums. This response to distress, in this instance a withdrawal, has become not only very pronounced, but also occurs following rather minimal provocation. (Photo 4.7)

Even smiles and cajoling from her "favorite" parent, Father, do not comfort her. (Photo 4.8)

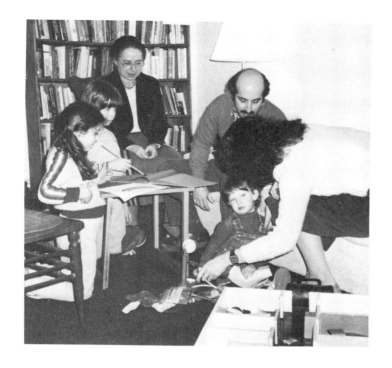

Photo 4.7

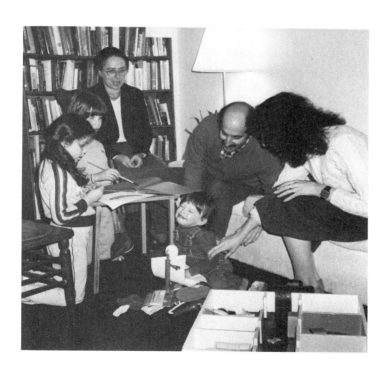

Photo 4.8

V. Whole Family Interaction

The alignment of intrafamilial alliances and divisions in this family can be seen clearly – Father and baby, Mother and middle daughter, and eldest, the identified patient, alone. The eldest, referred for problem behavior and obstinacy, remains isolated in many family interactions. (Photo 4.9)

In this picture, notice Mother's hands push away, directly toward the oldest child. This alignment and division were rigid, leaving the eldest in a deprived, pushed-away position in many whole family interactions. (Photo 4.10)

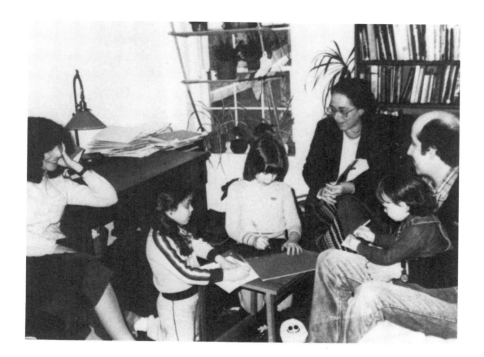

Photo 4.9

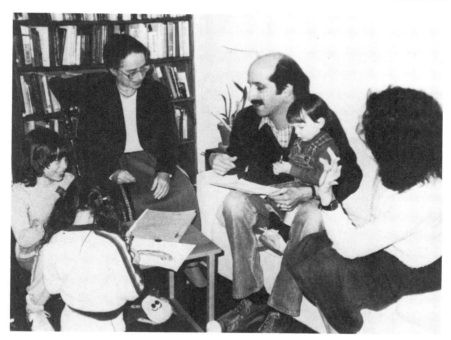

Photo 4.10

OBJECTIONS

The critical functions of young children in family therapy just described and depicted may have increased the theoretical understanding of the reader. Although recognition of these critical functions may now seem reasonable, objections are often immediately raised in practice by parents and therapist to the inclusion of younger children in family therapy endeavors. We will now discuss specifically 1) therapist objections, 2) parental objections, and 3) the objections of children themselves.

Therapist Objections

"I can't see children in my office!"

Including young children may present subjective difficulties to therapists who may express these troubles in seemingly objective or external concrete objections. Young children are seen as potential impediments to therapists' usual ways of conducting business. Therapists are accustomed to talking with adults and through this medium to produce "understanding," "insight," and improved "communication." Young children may be able to talk, but have a limited vocabulary, and incomplete understanding of abstract ideas. Children may be unable to sit through long sessions that contain mostly talk, and may become restless, and want to move around. This may be regarded as "a serious inconvenience" by the therapist. He or she may be willing or unwilling to modify his or her office and include play materials. (Some details of such modifications will be discussed in Chapter 7.)

Beyond concrete alterations and before making office changes, the therapist must be willing to face certain crucial questions within him- or herself. Will the young child be hurt by being included in unpleasant family confrontations in the office? What if the child learns secrets in the therapeutic sessions, from which he might otherwise have been ostensibly safely insulated and protected if left home?

After the therapist has decided to make the necessary minimal concrete and technical office modifications and answered the questions about confrontations, he or she may still carry the burden of overcoming other, inner resistances which are frequently experienced in a rationalized adult form: Children are too young, or too immature to understand or participate. But these are rationalizations − attempts to deal with the fact that it is not *easy* for some adults to relate naturally to children. They tend to either ignore children or to treat them with condescension that implies that children are incapable of serious and well-thought-out opinions of their own. And besides, children truly can be very trying!

Finally, as adults, therapists have had to renounce, in the course of their own development, the world of their childhood with varying degrees of reluctance; the danger to adult therapists of having childhood feelings and issues rearoused by including young children in family therapy is not to be discounted.

Parental Objections

> *"They will miss arithmetic class if they come to family therapy!"*

Parents, too, may raise objections. Frequently, these assume a practical or concrete form, e.g., the young children cannot miss school, Cub Scouts, or they will get home too late from therapy appointments. Underneath these objections, often not expressed directly, is the parents' wish to believe that they have done a good job as parents, and that their children, particularly those who are not obviously symptomatic, are "normal" and unscathed by family troubles. Parents are likely to feel inadequate and criticized by the recognition of problems. The inclusion of younger children may also be seen as pointing to larger, perhaps overwhelming problems. It is bad enough that they, or their older children, have "symptoms," but they would at least like to believe that they have raised other "healthy," younger children. The thought that all of their children may be affected by their family circumstances is frequently quite threatening to parents' self-esteem, since they feel they must be very poor parents. This form of resistance, when recognized by the therapist and discussed, is often approachable and resolvable.

When there is a "family secret," parental objections are frequently quite strong. And if, as is often the case, the parents are aware of their young children's ability to be outspoken, their objections will be even stronger. The establishment of safety and the use of tact and timing are most important. In the early stages of family treatment, therapists may use play materials to stop a premature revelation of a family secret by young children. Therapists may deliberately introduce the use of some material as a form of impediment to further discussion by its use at a time when the revelation of the family secret by children might disrupt, and even bring about premature termination of, family treatment.

Children's Objections

"My sister is nuts – not me."

Children themselves sometimes object, though less often than one might expect a priori, to family therapy. Indeed, the young child frequently has a fairly direct and intuitive grasp of parents' unvoiced feelings and is thus a good candidate as spokesperson for parental doubts and fears. The child may say, "Why do I have to be here? I am not the bad or weird one!" Frequently these doubts and fears are expressed in play or drawings as will be further described in the next chapter.

Given these many powerful objections, both internal and external, voiced and unvoiced, it is not surprising that many family therapists have preferred to treat "the whole family" without the presence of younger children. Indeed, there is a great deal of work that can be done with partial families, parents, and individuals. But, at times, we have experienced, in retrospect, paying a price for the exclusion of important young family members:

Many years ago, in a historically early case, we elected to see a family of two adolescent daughters and a retarded, much younger son, without the latter, who lived in a nearby school and came home regularly only on weekends. His inclusion was not considered or discussed. "Family" therapy progressed satisfactorily. But, follow-up five years later revealed a hitherto unexpressed, serious depression in Father. At that time both daughters were living out of the house. The father discussed serious, recurrent, depressive concerns about having no normal male "heir" in later life, issues that had not been approachable for discussion in the earlier family sessions. We speculated that these issues might have been treatable in the actual presence of the retarded young son "heir" who had been excluded by the therapists from family treatment.

In this chapter five critical functions of young children in family therapy have been defined and discussed:

1) tip of the iceberg;
2) beyond the tip;
3) allies and "co-therapists";
4) early detection; and
5) whole family interaction.

The previous five definitions and descriptions are not a complete list of critical functions within a family. There are other critical functions which centrally involve other family members in their operations. This list reflects the emphasis of this book on the critical functions of young children in family therapy.

In the following chapter, these critical functions will be amplified through further case descriptions and accompanying drawings.

CHAPTER NOTES

1) The term "critical function" of young children in family therapy has had a historically interesting progression. My early presentations and publications emphasized the use of play materials in family therapy (Zilbach, 1968). From this emphasis on play materials, I moved on to concentrate on young children (Zilbach, 1972). This increasing emphasis on children, particularly young children, enlarged and deepened, and was presented at a symposium on children in family therapy (Zilbach, 1977). Each of these steps represents my increasing understanding and conviction of the importance of whole families, and the particular critical functions of younger children in the practice of family therapy.

2) The "tip of the iceberg" critical function is an example of an expanded definition of function. This function was originally "young children as symptom-bearers." We realized that "symptom-bearing" was only one form of "tip," of access to the larger family problems that lie just below the surface, in the murky depths of the family, and so the function changed to its present state.

5

Illustrated Critical Functions

with Sharon Gordetsky

As stated in Chapter 1, this book has no hidden agenda, its message was stated at the outset. In the previous chapters one aspect has been emphasized, i.e., the necessity and importance of including young children in family therapy. The second aspect, play and the use of play materials, has been included but with less explicit emphasis. The photographs in Chapter 4 illustrate some use of play and play materials. In this chapter, the drawings which accompany the case vignettes illustrate in further detail the use of play materials, paper, and pen. There are other simple materials, such as clay, which are easily used for play but which are not described in this chapter.

Tip of the Iceberg

As has been discussed in Chapter 4, it frequently becomes a critical function of young children to call attention to trouble in their family. This is commonly accomplished through the formation of symptoms – "the tip of the iceberg" – the sign of underlying and much larger problems. The child who bears the presenting symptoms thus provides the "ticket of admission" to a potential source of help for the whole family:

> A family came to a community mental health clinic because
> the school principal threatened to suspend the "symptom-bearer,"
> a 10-year-old boy, unless the family sought psychological treat-

Sharon Gordetsky, Ph.D., is Chief Psychologist, Parents' and Children's Services, Boston, Massachusetts.

ment. The youngster had been having increasing difficulty completing work assignments in school and had gotten into many fights with teachers and peers, kicking and cursing them for no outwardly apparent reason. The family was upset by the referral, denying the existence of any similar difficulties at home or anywhere else.

During an initial family interview, this youngster and his younger sibling sat close to each other, both drawing quietly while the parents voiced their annoyance at the school and their confusion about the recommendation for mental health intervention. About 20 minutes into the first interview, the therapist asked the children about their drawings. In one of them (see Drawing 5.1), the 10-year-old depicted a house, a tree, and clouds typical of many drawings of latency-age children. However, of particular interest to the therapist was the large, looming, black tornado and a tiny stick figure tucked into the window calling for "help." "What kind of help," the therapist asked, "does the person in the window want?" The therapist put his finger directly on the stick figure. "He's so scared," the boy explained, "he doesn't know how to stop the storms around the house." This simple, clear, and poignant message provided the first opportunity to openly discuss the marital discord and frequent "stormy" fights that occurred at home.

Now the therapist was able to help the parents more easily recognize and understand the significance of their son's "stormy" behavior in the classroom, despite his "good" behavior at home. Without the impetus of the 10-year-old's behavior, his "symptoms," and the "storms" at school, these parents might never have sought counseling. They had not been aware of how their "stormy" quarreling at home – only a part of their marital troubles – was affecting their child.

Beyond the Tip of the Iceberg

The explicit recognition of the troubles or symptoms contained in the "tip of the iceberg" may tempt clinicians to limit their vision. As discussed in the previous chapter, the "identified patient" may actually be the healthiest family member. Just beyond "the tip," the obvious symptoms, may be even more serious pain and pathology in some other member of the family, or more global severe family dysfunction:

72   Drawing 5.1

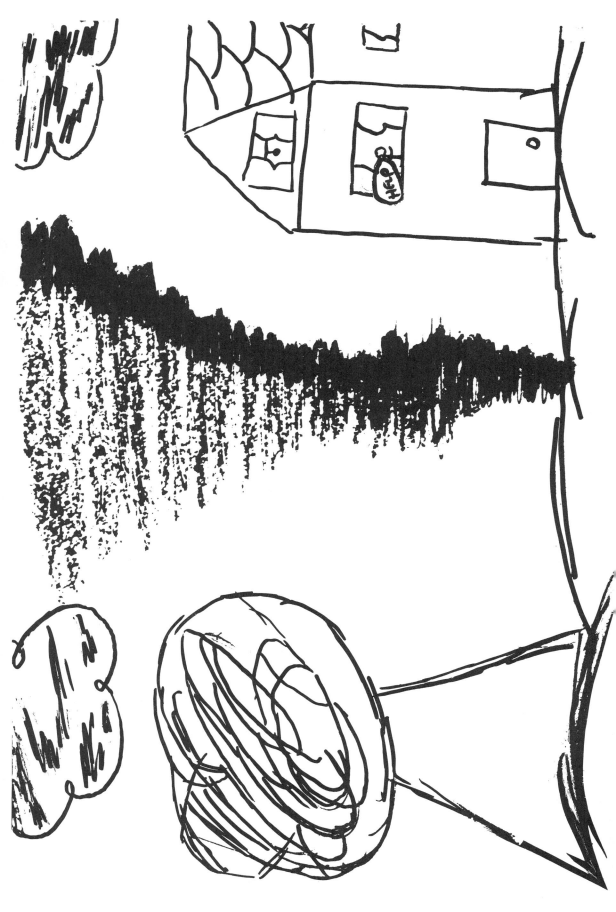

A seven-year-old with daytime and nighttime enuresis was referred for evaluation. Her school performance was adequate and her teacher viewed her socially as "active, but well-adjusted." At the suggestion of the family pediatrician, the mother, a concerned middle-class, professional woman, requested a psychological evaluation. In the individual evaluation interviews, the child was a likable, precocious youngster who played actively (Note 1). Throughout the family meeting her asymptomatic, "normal," eight-year-old sister worked on the drawing reproduced in Drawing 5.2: a female face clearly demarcated in heavy black, surrounded by dark purple scribbling, with piercing eyes, and a gaping, screaming mouth. The girls, who often playacted in sessions, were asked to make up and enact a story about this picture. One youngster pretended to be "a mother who just screamed and cried, screamed and cried." The girls' mother, who usually remained controlled but often seemed annoyed, began to weep. Only then did she tell the therapist how depressed and overwhelmed she felt, and that she didn't know if she had the energy or patience to take care of her children. The children, worried about their mother who had previously been "taken away" to a mental hospital, used their drawings and play to communicate their fear to the therapist and to aid their mother in asking for the help she needed.

For many reasons, children cannot easily talk directly about themselves or other members of their family. Similarly, they often may have trouble admitting they are upset or worried – believing that their parents wish them to be happy and secure. Therapists interviewing children understandably feel frustrated when children do not seem to pay attention or answer their questions in words. However, children often can "talk" more easily about themselves and others through play and drawings, and in this way provide important information and insights that therapists seek:

A separated mother and her four children agreed to a family evaluation, although only one child was currently having "trouble" in school. The children talked about missing their father and wanting their mother to let them see him more. The mother had a hard time in the interviews and frequently just sat and cried. The therapist made direct suggestions about increasing the father's visitations which Mother adamantly refused to do. The therapist felt frustrated

Drawing 5.2

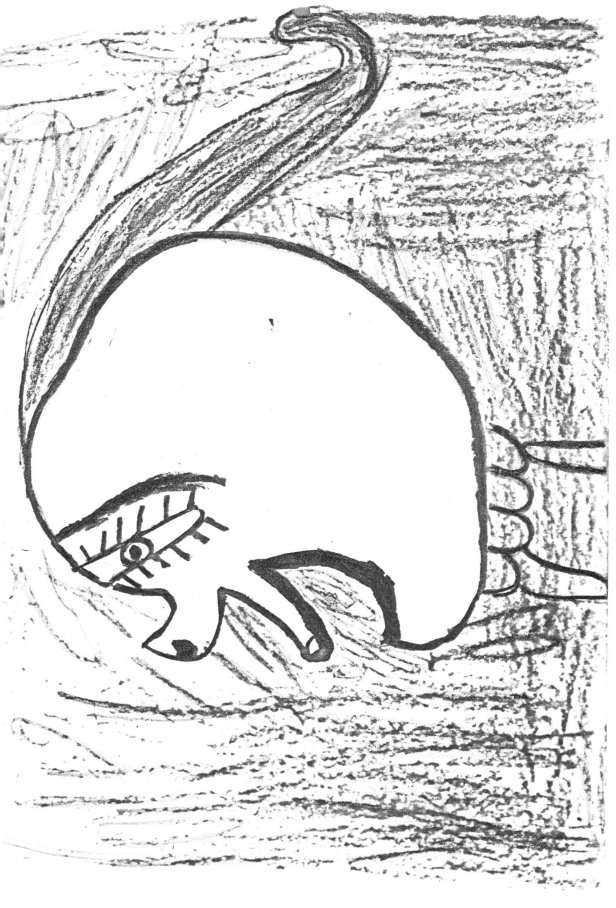

at this mother's seeming insensitivity in not allowing her children more contact with their father. During a family interview, the therapist noticed one of the children creating a comic strip (Drawing 5.3) and asked him to share it with the family. The drawing showed a superhero – "Super Duh" – coming to the rescue of a frightened figure being held at gunpoint. As the assailant is overcome he says, "I give up." In the same frame, our hero "Super Duh" shouts "Fa duh" and then flys away. An important message about wanting the family meetings to continue was communicated to the therapist by the child's statement in writing below the final frame, "stayed tuned for the next issue."

During the next session, the therapist reminded the boy that she was promised another episode of "Super Duh." Only then did mother and son report to the therapist and the other family members that, during a previous visit, the father had pointed a gun at the mother and threatened to shoot her. This son, the creator of the comic strip, had been the only witness. This incident remained a secret between them, but a secret that they did not speak about even with each other, until this family meeting. There is a pointing gun in Frame 4 of "Super Duh." The other children and the therapist could now understand their mother's anxiety about their father's visits, and the "identified patient" no longer needed to safeguard his and his mother's secret. Almost immediately following this session, the boy's school problems abated.

Allies and "Co-therapists"

As explained in Chapter 4, children frequently function as allies of the therapist, and sometimes as "co-therapists," in the therapeutic process. They can express, either verbally or through play and behavior, essential family themes and feelings. Although a therapist might be cognizant of such family issues or feelings, it may be difficult for the therapist alone to bring them to the surface to be explored in the therapy sessions. It is in these instances that children, as therapeutic allies, often lend a helping hand:

> For many weeks, when the G family came to family therapy sessions, the parents angrily attacked the oldest of these three young boys for being lazy and irresponsible and "clipping" small items that didn't belong to him. Since they often bought him, without ques-

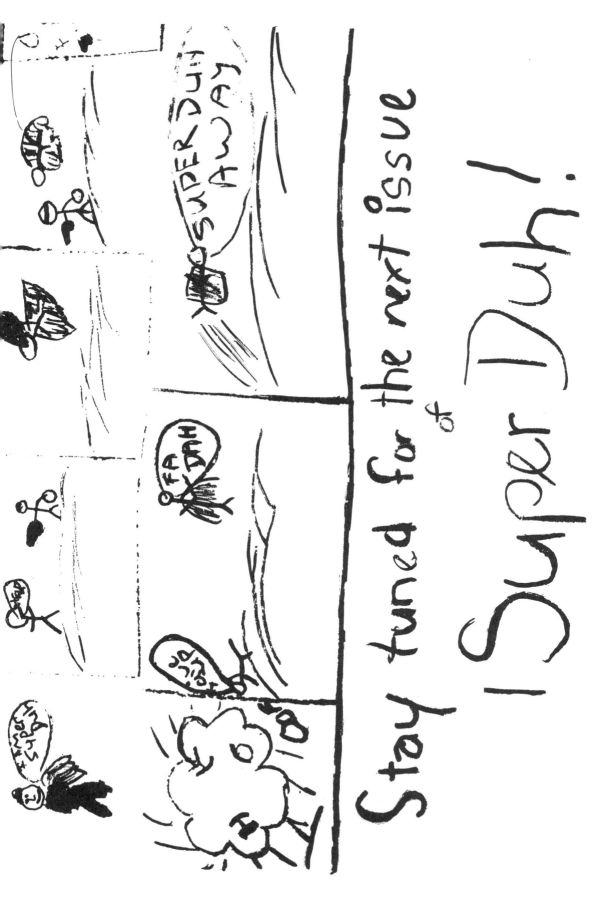

Stay tuned for the next issue of ¡Super Duh!

tion, many big and small things, his behavior angered them. The large amount of supplies the children used and their constant seeking of her attention quickly alerted the therapist to the sadness and emotional deprivation of this family. However, a direct statement or interpretation about this by the therapist would likely have been met with denial and resistance since, as they remarked at least once in each meeting, "Despite his 'clipping,' our children are really good, and everything else in our family is fine."

However, then the oldest of these "good" boys produced a drawing of an armless, shapeless, listless boy lying on his bed in a vacant room (see Drawing 5.4). The messages and feelings evoked by this drawing, which the child had not expressed in words, could be examined by the family and the therapist together. The parents saw how empty and lonely their son depicted himself, alone in his room, which, in reality, was filled with many toys and games. By the end of this session, the parents and children began using the therapy hour candidly to discuss family conflicts concerning alcoholism and the large amount of time the parents spent away from home. The children described their parents' time away from home as "going out to parties to drink booze," leaving the boys feeling very alone, neglected, and upset.

In addition to making accessible crucial family facts or themes, children can ally themselves with the treatment process in other ways. In the following example, the therapist's ability to form a positive relationship with the children was critical to overcoming the mother's resistance to continuing family therapy:

After two weeks of participating in a family diagnostic evaluation, Mrs. H began speaking of her reluctance to continue, despite her knowledge that her daughter was in serious danger of failing in school. As Mrs. H spoke of the great inconvenience and time involved in the therapy appointments, her 13-year-old daughter drew a picture of a farm scene ravaged by an erupting volcano and a cloudburst. The rain or tears, the windstorm, and the exploding volcano all represented the feelings the girl was unable to express to her mother (see Drawing 5.5 on p. 81). However, using the drawing as a springboard, the therapist encouraged the daughter to tell her mother how upset she felt. The mother had no notion

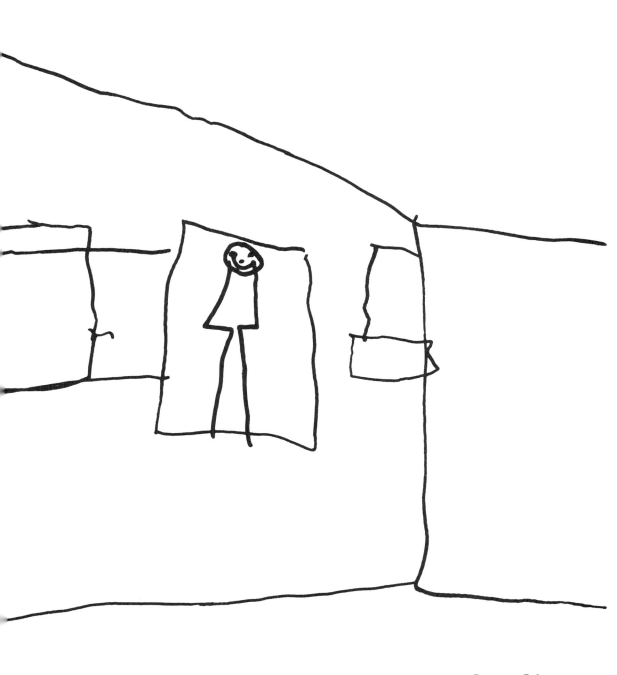

Drawing 5.4

of how troubled her daughter was; she had only known about how badly the daughter behaved. In this case, the girl's sadness and distress, as depicted in the drawings, and her confidence in the family therapy (the tears also represented her sadness at the mother's wish to stop the treatment), motivated the mother to continue. The message in the picture, which illustrated how much this child needed and wanted help, was more powerful than the therapist's recommendation.*

Children as Early Detectors

Family therapy provides practitioners with the opportunity to meet and evaluate all family members. As discussed in the section entitled "Beyond the Tip of the Iceberg," we have found that frequently the most needy member of a family is not "the identified patient." In other instances, we have seen family members who are currently symptom-free but who, without some form of intervention, are likely to experience difficulties in the future.

In the following case example, the therapist's insistence that all the children attend the therapy session brought early attention to a psychosomatic symptom that might otherwise have gone undetected and led to more serious physical and psychological sequelae:

The J family came seeking help for three of their four children. Their only "normal, happy" child, the youngest daughter, came eagerly to sessions with the rest of her family. She always smiled and appeared to be quietly happy and well-adjusted, exactly as her parents described her. Throughout early sessions, her parents held her up as an example to their other children. However, during one family treatment hour, this child drew a well-formed sea creature with a hanging belly; she colored the creature black but left a small, yet distinct, hole inside the belly. She then, with the help of an older "retarded" sibling, labeled the creature "meshuga," which means "crazy" in Yiddish (see Drawing 5.6 on p. 83). The "retarded" sister, who in actuality had a severe learning disability, pointed to the hole. "Look at that," she yelled. The therapist turned to the picture, remarking that it looked like a fish with a big belly. The thera-

---

*Drawing 5.5 was produced by an adolescent, rather than a young child. However, the message was drawn so powerfully that the author felt it was useful to include in this book.

Drawing 5.5

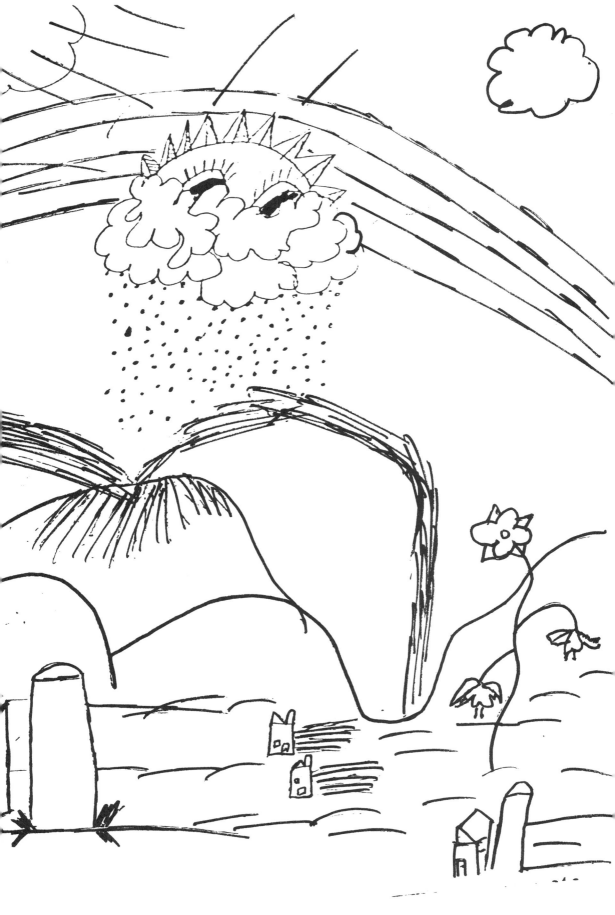

pist wondered aloud about the hole, finally guessing that such a hole might give the sea creature stomachaches. "I have a stomachache," the young child-artist volunteered. The therapist then asked this usually quiet child to describe her symptoms, which had started seriously two weeks earlier. The parents confessed they had known nothing about the stomachaches because "she never complains." Shortly thereafter, this girl was diagnosed as actually having a stomach ulcer.

The family's expectation that this child remain "good" and trouble-free was clear to her. The implicit requirement to be "normal" prevented her from directly complaining about her physical symptoms either at home or in therapy. She had learned, however, that the therapist always looked at all the artwork, whether produced by the "patients" or the "normal child." So she chose this safer way of "complaining" about her stomach pains and was ably assisted by her sister's shout, "Look at that!" The "hole in the belly" drawing, and the parents' surprise at this child's hesitancy to complain, provided the therapist with the opportunity to explore the rigid "good-normal" versus "bad-retarded/sick" dichotomy that had evolved in this family.

In another case, the inclusion of an asymptomatic six-year-old boy in family therapy led to the probable prevention of a severe childhood depression. As in the previous case and numerous others, the asymptomatic child was represented as "perfect, a delight, never any trouble." And, during early family meetings, he indeed always was perfectly behaved. In fact, until the therapist actively engaged him, encouraging him to use the play materials and to speak when he wished, he sat silently and was ignored totally by the other family members. This was especially true because the parents wanted to spend all of the treatment time talking about their older daughter, who was constantly in trouble.

These parents initially objected to play materials being used at all during the session. They complained that the children were not there to have fun and that play materials would be a distraction to important discussions. However, this young child quietly drew many pictures from the beginning of the initial family evaluation session, and, over time, his parents became more accepting of the use of play materials. The drawings were typical drawings of houses, or of the child and his dog playing. But slowly, his drawings began to change in content. The safe environment of the family meetings, and his growing awareness that the therapist paid attention to him, allowed him to

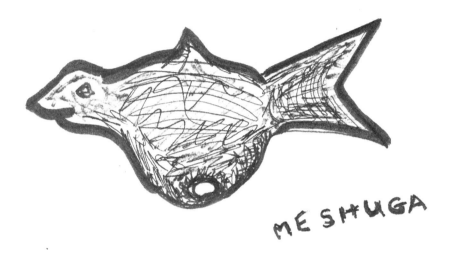

MESHUGA

Drawing 5.6

participate fully in the therapy through his drawings. In one of them (Drawing 5.7), the black background, the sad expression, including the tears which ran right into the message "Oh rain," were important clues about this young child's underlying feelings of depression and his readiness to begin to let his parents know about these feelings.

Using this younger boy's pictures as a starting point, the therapist could easily direct some attention to him. Direct exploration of Drawing 5.7 and similar drawings ("Can you tell your parents why you feel so bad?") led to cries from the child about how neglected and hated he felt: "You (the parents) wish I wasn't born. . . . You spend all your time with R (another sibling) and never say anything to me. . . . " Once these pictures introduced this child's feelings of neglect and deprivation into the therapy sessions, the parents were able to recognize how they confused his being "good" with not needing them. Only then did the parents acknowledge their feelings and subsequently were able to rearrange their lives in order to meet this child's needs in a more complete and satisfactory fashion. In addition, refocusing the attention away from the "identified patient" proved beneficial for him as well.

Whole Family Interactions: The Dynamics and Quality of Whole Family Understanding

As discussed earlier in Chapter 4 on the critical functions of young children in family therapy, in order for a therapist to appreciate how any family functions or dysfunctions s/he needs to see all family members, including the very youngest, together over a period of time. Children often communicate fundamental family conditions that shape both family and individual development, as well as illustrate, via their behavior, play, words and affects, the way the family functions as a whole unit:

> The K family consulted a child therapist seeking help for their five-year-old son, who had bad temper outbursts. As part of the routine diagnostic procedure, a family interview was held that included the other two children, an eight-year-old son and a three-year-old daughter. The two older children were unusually quiet and sedentary for their ages. They did not attempt any exploration of the play materials in the office, although these were abundant and clearly in view. In fact, these youngsters would leave their jackets on and closed tightly for an entire session if they were not given direct, concrete parental permission to open and remove

Drawing 5.7

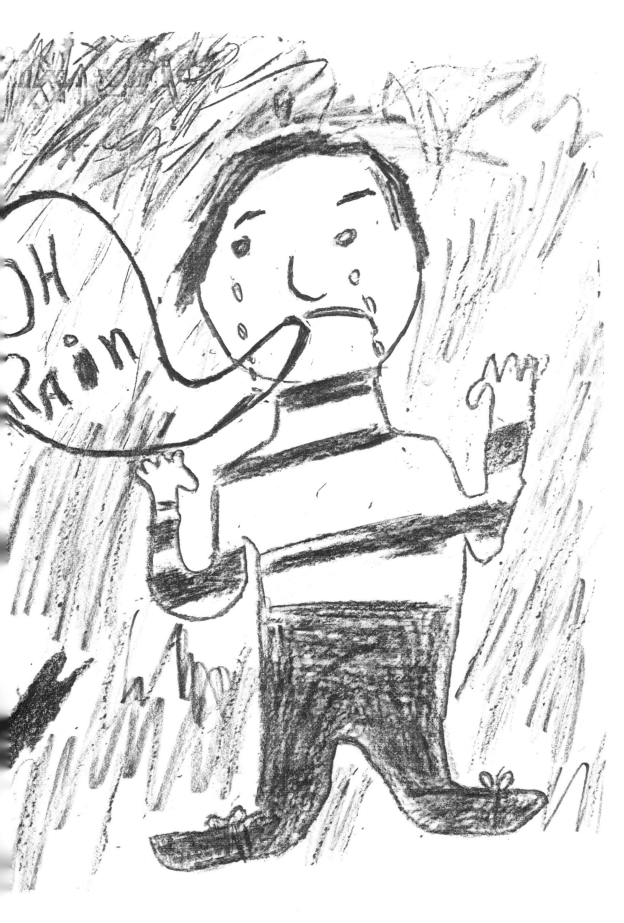

them. Only the youngest, the three-year-old comfortably wandered around, busily dumping toys from an old toy box, interrupting with questions and requests for help from her mother.

Both older boys were very polite and cooperative, and initially refused the therapist's offer to draw or play if they wished. They often responded to the therapist's or their parents' verbal questioning by minimally shrugging their shoulders. However, when regular family meetings were proposed, as part of the therapy recommendations, all three children appeared eager to participate.

During the initial phase of family treatment, the therapist actively sought a way to help the children communicate in the sessions. Although the parents preferred that the children "speak out if they have something to say," the therapist recognized that the boys were too anxious. She reiterated and emphasized her permission to use the play materials, explaining that it might help them feel less nervous in the session, and added that some children like to draw and play the things they think about. In addition, she encouraged the parents to give their permission for the children to use the materials.

The therapist tried, through play and drawings, to reach the hidden aspects of the children's personalities and of the family. The children began slowly and tentatively to draw pictures and soon were producing many pictures during each session. Drawings allowed them to continue to be quiet and obedient, while simultaneously providing an effective and affective avenue of expression. The older boy, who had not been referred, began to produce many pictures similar to Drawing 5.8. Each drawing in this series contained big "sharks with sharp teeth trying to catch and swallow the little fish." After a time, puppet shows were being produced about dangerous, underwater sharks with "big, sharp teeth that scared and hurt the little fish even in its own (fish) family."

This particular theme of danger and fear in the family was depicted so frequently, and with such intensity and apparent purposefulness, that it alerted the therapist to the need for further exploration into the "shark" family situation. (Note in Drawing 5.8 the very sharp, black teeth and the fiery tongue lashing out of the big fish's mouth. The small fish were never drawn with teeth or open mouths.) Examining these drawings in family sessions, the therapist wondered with the family why there were so many pictures of small fish be-

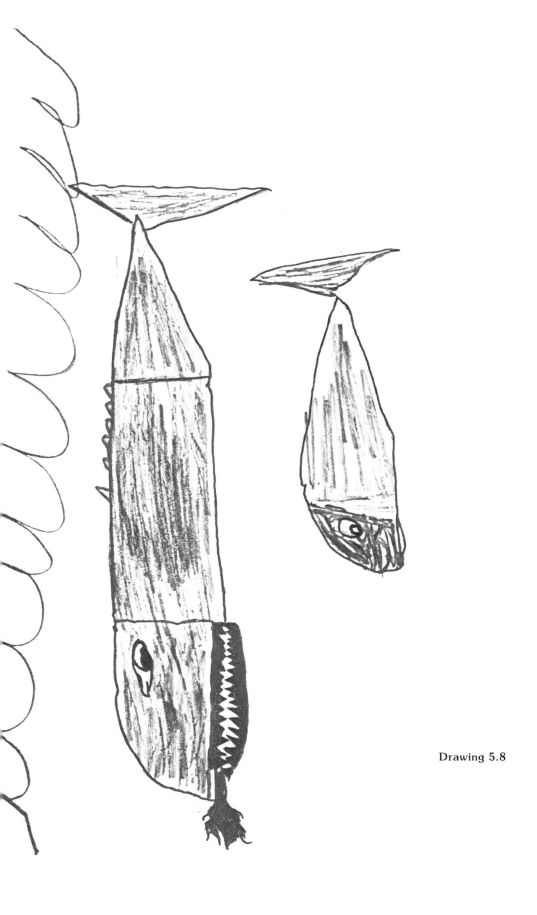

Drawing 5.8

ing frightened and hurt. Only then did the mother voice feelings consistent with her son's drawings. She explained that their house was indeed a frightening place due to the father's unpredictable outbursts, which frequently resulted in the children being physically hurt. In this case, the children's drawings and puppet shows expressed their previously unspoken feelings of fear about their father. Their play finally brought these "secrets" into treatment and enabled a fuller understanding of the family atmosphere and relationships.

In this chapter each of the critical functions of including young children in family therapy has been illustrated by case vignettes and drawings. The pictures and case material vividly portray that the inclusion of young children is not only useful, but often necessary for family therapy.

CHAPTER NOTE

1) When an individual child with symptoms is referred, a full diagnostic evaluation includes both individual and family interviews. It is most important to establish, at the outset, that family interviews are part of the regular diagnostic series.

6

A Family in Treatment: Selected Themes and Drawings

with Sharon Gordetsky and David Brown

In the last chapter, brief vignettes from several families and accompanying drawings illustrated the critical functions young children may serve in family treatment. In this chapter, we will focus our discussion on one family whom we will call the Roberts. The children in this family play and draw in their family therapy sessions in order to communicate family issues that might otherwise remain underground, or at least take much longer to be raised by the adults. It is not the purpose of this chapter to present a complete case study, nor to present all of the family data, therapeutic strategies, or treatment outcome. Rather, the purpose is to illustrate concretely and specifically the unfolding of family themes, family conflicts, and struggles, through the play and drawings of two children.

As has been discussed in previous chapters, play, not abstract ideas or concepts, is the natural language of young children. Through this mode children communicate what is important to them. Often, young children may not "know" in cognitive terms what underlying conflicts or issues are upsetting them.

Sharon Gordetsky, Ph.D., is Chief Psychologist, Parents' and Children's Services, Boston, Massachusetts. David Brown, M.D., is Senior Staff Physician, Pediatrics and Psychiatry, Children's Hospital Medical Center, Boston, Massachusetts; and Instructor, Harvard Medical School, Cambridge, Massachusetts.

But, affectively, they do "know" and, when given the opportunity, they can express themselves. The pictures and play produced by the two children in the Roberts family reveal the family climate and central family themes that the parents may not have been aware of or might have preferred not to discuss.

The children used their drawings and play to tell the team of male and female co-therapists about themselves and their family. They also used play to cope with their inevitable anxiety during stressful moments in the therapy sessions. One can see in the development of these pictures both the expressive and defensive functions of play as described and defined in Chapters 2, 3, and 4.

The Roberts family came to family treatment with a specific goal, stated by the Father: to help the family negotiate the transition from a nuclear, one-home, two-parent, two-child, one-pet family to a separated and divorced family living in two homes in different parts of a city. Thus, family division and separation was a central issue for the family – both internally and interpersonally. Also, as one might suspect, not all members agreed with the Father's main agenda, and those who did not frequently used treatment as a vehicle for expressing other equally important family concerns and problems.

The Roberts family consisted of two parents who had been married for 18 years and their two children: Eric, 10, and Jenny, six. Treatment was initiated by the father after an abrupt and rapid separation. Immediately after the separation, the mother had moved the children from their former home to a distant city in another part of the country. Mr. Roberts convinced his wife to return to his city so he could pursue a stable relationship with his children. In addition, he hoped that therapy would provide the opportunity for the parents to work toward a more amicable divorce. The mother hesitantly cooperated, but the children were clearly relieved to see the family together again in the family sessions.

The parents, both middle-aged and intelligent, came from very different backgrounds; they met when the father was in Italy with the Marine Corps. They married and moved to the United States where, after 10 years of trying to conceive, they decided to adopt children. Both children were young infants at the time of their adoption. The parents, who were devoted to their children and delighted to have them, assumed fairly conventional roles of housekeeper and breadwinner, wherein mother stayed at home doing much of the child care and father held an executive position. As previously mentioned, their marital separation was abrupt, and both parents were left feeling angry and disappointed in each other.

When the co-therapists, a male-female team, first met with the Roberts family the room seemed flooded with emotion. Besides the anger and resentment that made everyone uncomfortable, there was Mrs. Roberts' deep hurt about the circumstances surrounding her separation from her husband. The children, both bright, active, and engaging, were simultaneously relieved to see their father and extremely anxious about the separation and planned divorce. Clearly, their wish was to reunite the family, which was compatible with their mother's hidden agenda at the beginning of treatment, to be reunited with her husband.

The parents agreed to meet weekly with the team of two family therapists and to bring both of their children to the sessions. From the outset, the children spontaneously used the play material they found in the therapy room, and incorporated the office furniture and blackboard into their activities. Throughout the treatment, which lasted approximately 15 months, the children produced drawings that chronicled the feelings and conflicts in the family. It was primarily through their drawings that the children were able to participate in treatment most comfortably.

As one would expect, the therapy went through various phases, and several major themes developed, not all centered on the planned divorce. These themes reflected interpersonal relationships within the family, as well as the children's perceptions of themselves.

For purposes of illustration, the children's drawings have been placed into four major categories: 1) the children's view of family therapy; 2) the separation and divorce; 3) the children's view of the marital and child-parent relationship; and 4) the children's messages about themselves (Note 1).

Each picture has specific elements which are direct communications from the children to the therapists and/or to their parents. Sometimes these are embodied in labels or messages written on the pictures, sometimes in the construction of the drawings, or sometimes in the use of the materials, e.g., both sides of a single sheet to present both sides of a dilemma. Throughout, messages are transmitted in terms of both subjects depicted and colors used. The following discussions of the pictures will point out what the therapists noticed, the picture's likely significance, and what was happening concurrently in the family and in the treatment.

THE CHILDREN'S VIEW OF FAMILY THERAPY

During the beginning weeks of treatment, Jenny drew many flower pictures typical of drawings by latency-age children (early elementary school). She drew these flowers both as self-expression, and as a way of making things look pretty and happy, for indeed this was her main role in the family. Drawing 6.1

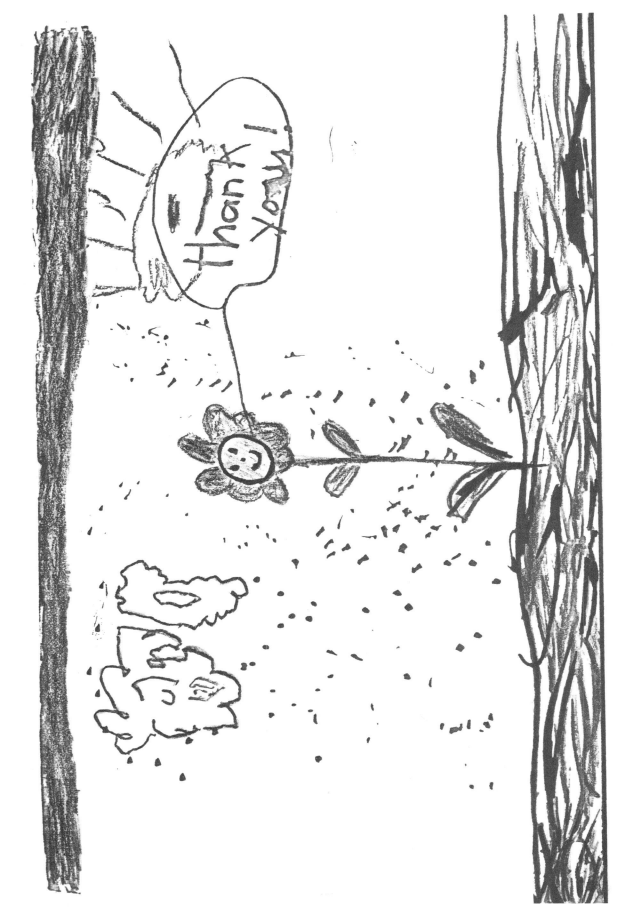

is different from her earlier flower drawings in several ways. The typical bright yellow sun on the right that had appeared in many earlier pictures, here evolves into yellow rain clouds on the left. The isolated flower, with a face exclaiming Jenny's thanks to the therapists, is related to her expressed wish that the therapy help her parents reunite; the rain is the first outward expression of Jenny's sadness and wish to cry. Recognizing the significance of this drawing, and particularly its differences from previous drawings, the therapists drew the family's attention to it. Jenny was then able to talk about her hopes for the family and about her own sad feelings and unhappiness.

Jenny's role in her family was to be strong, competent, and happy. Although she was younger than her brother, she was physically stronger and did much better in school than Eric, who was encopretic and immature. This image of Jenny as the bearer of positive affect and as a caretaker consistently appears in her drawings. In Drawing 6.2, however, a drawing made in the only session her parents did not attend, Jenny depicts herself as a smiling little girl in the therapy room, comfortably seated in a big chair near a play-table full of toys. Here we see the appearance of more organized, age-appropriate latency material. There is less evidence of overwhelming feelings than in drawings done in other sessions. In this picture, made as a gift for the female therapist, Jenny was telling the therapists what it was like for her to be in treatment with adults with whom she could be a little girl working and playing, rather than bearing the burden of being the overcompetent member of this unhappy family.

THE SEPARATION AND DIVORCE

Early in treatment, Jenny drew a picture of herself playing with the family dog (Drawing 6.3). Once again many features of this drawing are typical. The child and dog are smiling, the sun is shining, and flowers are blooming. Of particular note, however, is the large size of the dog's house, the heavy black and red smoke pouring from the chimney, and the sad face drawn on the largest flower, which stands out from the rest. This was the first time a pet had been mentioned, and both children eagerly told the therapists about their dog, who no longer lived with them as it had been given away at the time of the separation. When Jenny was questioned about her drawing, she described a big fire in the fireplace (which we could not see, although the door was bright red) that might burn up the dog's house. The discussion that followed, which turned to fond memories of the past, including the dog, allowed the children to ventilate their fears of destruction and loss.

Drawing 6.1

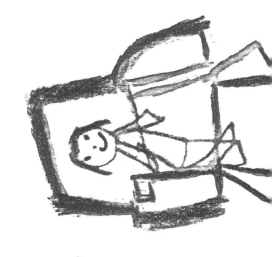

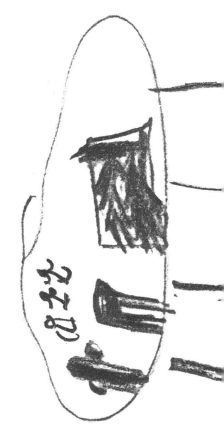

Drawing 6.2

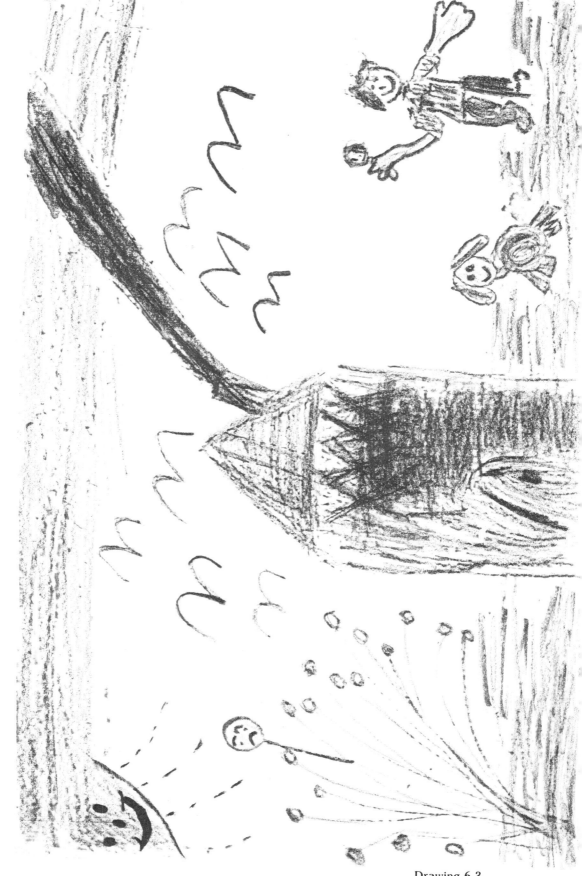

Drawing 6.3

This was the first time that either child had drawn a house or the dog, and this drawing was of a house and a dog that no longer existed for them. When the therapists made this observation, the parents disclosed their recent discussions about housing options. The father wanted his wife and children to have a house, while he would rent an apartment for himself. Mother did not agree with Father's ideas. That such a concrete and seemingly final plan was being discussed caused great anxiety in the children, because they had not been part of these "house" discussions outside the therapy session. Thus, this first drawing of house and dog precipitated a first discussion of housing plans with the children.

During the same family session in which Jenny produced Drawing 6.3, her brother drew a scene of two people on bicycles about to collide (Drawing 6.4). As noted above, Jenny's picture prompted her parents to discuss their conflicts about housing. During this discussion Eric sat busily drawing. In Drawing 6.4 two male bicyclists are facing each other. One bicyclist, Eric said, "is zooming down the hill and is gonna crash into the other guy." The scene of the crash is a messily colored brown mound, an encopretic image that was repeated in many pictures. Eric's anger at his perfectionist father is symbolized by the collision of the two males, and his conflict around alliances was clearly enacted by his uncertainty about which parent to give his picture to.

Both children frequently gave their drawings as gifts to their parents. The dilemma of which parent to give a picture to is often present for young children, but for these children it was a very difficult choice – as is evidenced in this picture by Eric's first writing "mommy" and adding just underneath "daddy." When the therapists asked the children about this, they admitted it was hard to decide because their parents couldn't share the drawings as they used to. Then the children voiced in some detail their sadness about the divorce, something that the parents were unable to do for a long time.

After giving his father the picture of the bicyclists, Eric returned to the playtable and resumed drawing. The therapists wondered out loud if this next drawing would be for his mother, since he had just made a gift to his father. Eric did not answer in words, but continued to concentrate on his artwork. Spurred on by his previous drawing, Eric now showed even more dramatically, and with less inhibition, his feelings and fears.

Whereas the crash was anticipated in Drawing 6.4, the big, loud crash ("Boom") in Drawing 6.5 takes place in the center of chaos. The "boom" is a collision of brown and green crayon markings. Similarly, all the opposing figures are either brown or green. Frightened figures are crying "help!" and "watch out," while other figures are being destroyed and flung into the air.

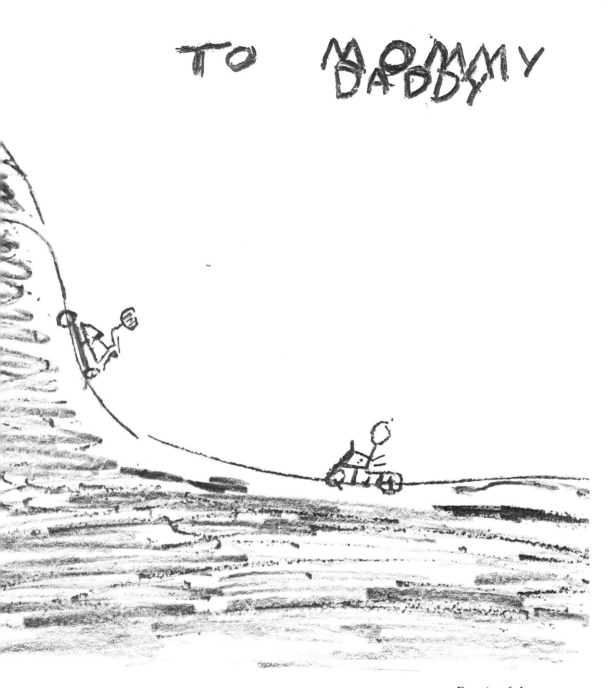

Drawing 6.4

We see for the first time in this drawing a conflict between the browns and the greens. This battle scene and theme, brown versus green, was depicted frequently in many different versions from then on throughout the course of the therapy. The therapists understood the brown versus green theme as symbolizing Eric's struggles with his father. The child represented himself in fecal brown, and his dejected and angry facial expressions symbolized his low self-esteem, as well as his parents' concern about his encopresis. Eric drew his father in Marine green – the color Father wore when Mother first met him.

Pictures such as Drawing 6.5 made a serious impact on the other family members. Eric, who was usually a quiet boy, rarely expressed his anxiety to his parents verbally. The loud cries for "help" in the pictures, however, could not be ignored. By the end of this session, the parents jointly acknowledged their children's messages for help. Thereafter, Mr. and Mrs. Roberts were better able to openly discuss their housing and other dilemmas with their children's best interests in mind.

As time passed, and the initial fantasies about how therapy would reunite the family faded, arguments between the parents increased and the children grew more upset. Drawings 6.6 and 6.7, two sides of one deliberately torn sheet of paper, were drawn when, after some months of separation, the impending divorce was discussed more openly. The anxiety and uncertainty about where people would live was more evident and openly expressed. Like the family, Drawings 6.6 and 6.7 are partly split down the middle. On the left side of Drawing 6.6, Eric drew a sun and labeled it in yellow, the only bright color on this side of the page. However, directly opposite the sun is a cloud labeled in black. Once again Eric drew a house and clearly placed his family's name next to it. This house, no longer a happy memory, is drawn in heavy black and, representing the original family house, is under a cloud. Every element in the drawing is carefully labeled, "grass, bark, leves (leaves)," including such things as would ordinarily go unseen such as "roots." In addition, an arrow points to each object to ensure that there can be no misunderstanding. The house is labeled twice (note the arrow). This compulsive, concrete labeling is a direct response to Eric's anxiety about the breaking up of his family.

On the reverse side of the picture, which shows a big, stable tree with its roots being split in half, Eric drew his house, no longer whole but similarly torn apart (Drawing 6.7). His response to this separation is clear. He portrays himself as a prostrated, helpless child crying for help to an unidentified, robot-like figure next to him. He colors his body red, signifying how full of strong feeling he is, in spite of his quiet outward demeanor. He gives himself no hands,

Drawing 6.5

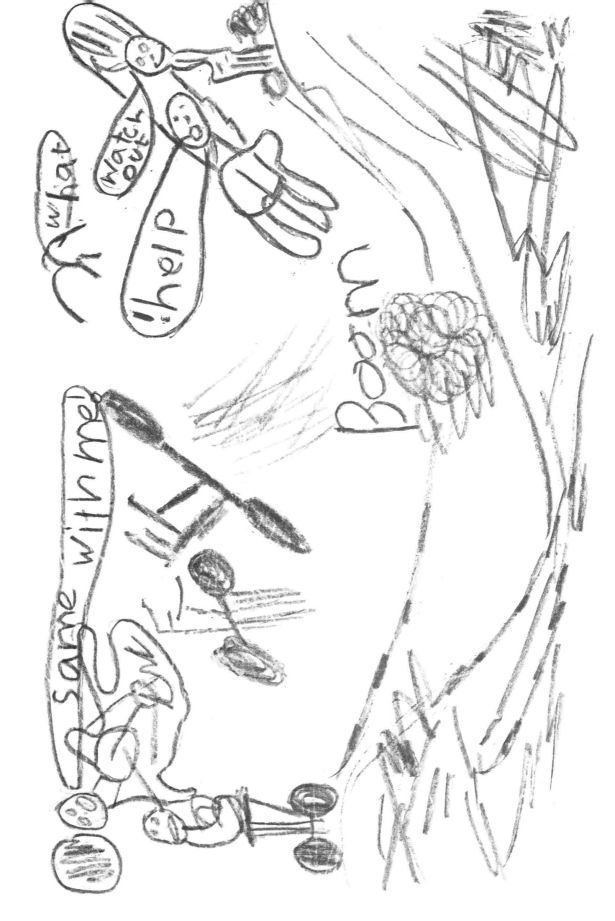

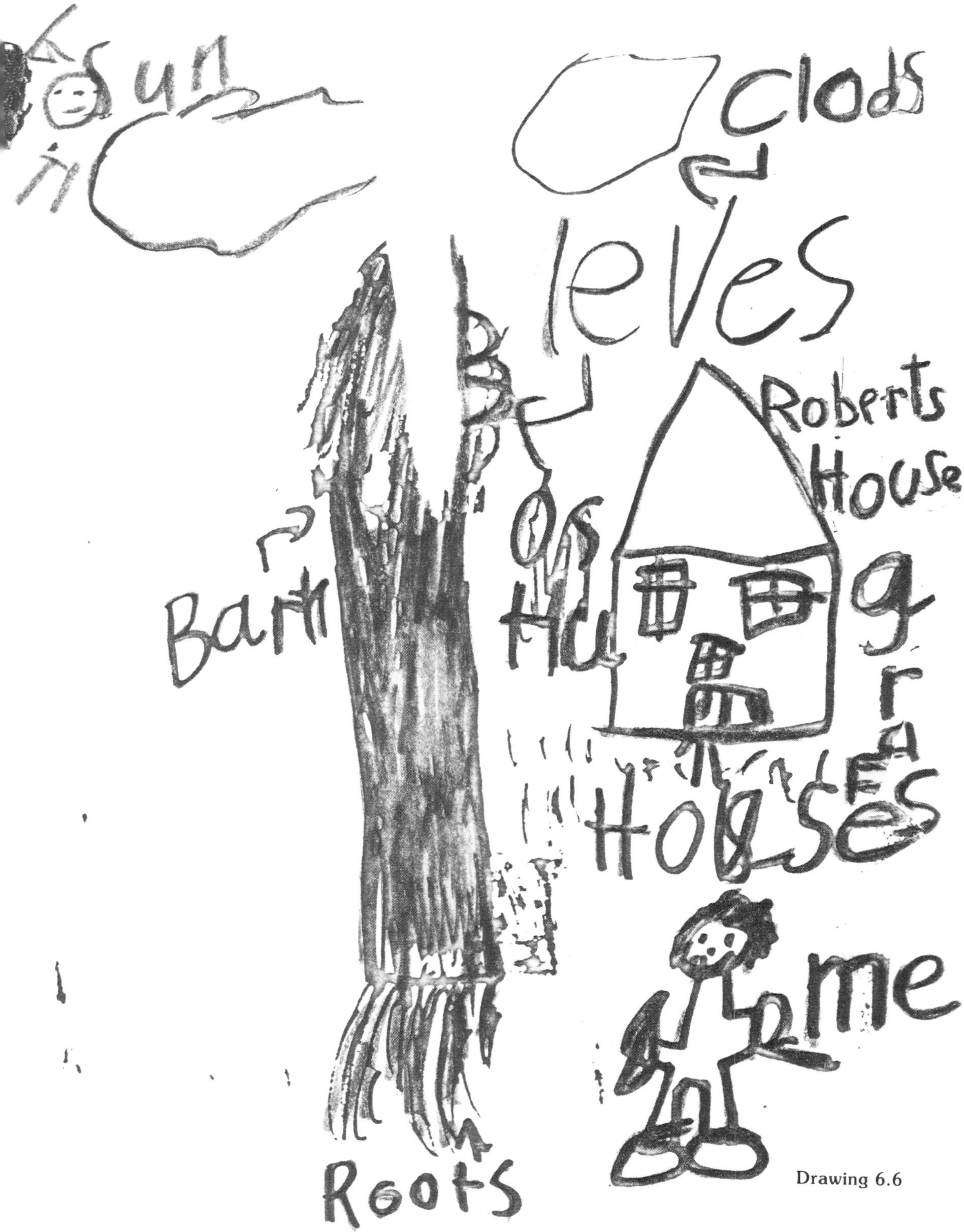

Sun

clods

leves

Roberts House

Bark

Hu

grases

Houses

me

Roots

Drawing 6.6

To: Mc AMy

From: Eric

Drawing 6.7

although from previous drawings, we know he is capable of drawing hands and fingers. He also draws himself in a spread-eagle posture, indicating how torn and defeated he feels.

It is interesting to compare Drawings 6.6 and 6.7 to the earlier picture of the house, boy, and dog (see Drawing 6.3). Although the red and black smoke pouring from the chimney in the earlier drawing (Drawing 6.3) indicates that there is much smoldering going on behind the closed doors, the earlier, more cheerful outdoor scene suggests that the amount of anxiety about the family is significantly less than it was when the later drawings (Drawings 6.6 and 6.7) were produced.

How were these drawings useful in the family treatment? They communicated to everyone in the therapy room how anxious and angry the children were about their parents' fights and divorce plans. The children felt overwhelmed by the chaos, and too frightened and incompetent to influence their parents' behavior. But the therapists were able to use the children's drawings to show the parents dramatically and concretely how their children were being affected by their arguments. Since both parents wanted what was best for their children, and since their stated purpose for seeking therapy was to negotiate a more amicable divorce and joint custody arrangement, the drawings pushed them to see that their constant bickering was making their children feel overwhelmed and torn apart. Some therapists might have been hesitant to include such young children in "parents' business." However, despite the intense discomfort of some of the family meetings, these therapists felt that, if the children were not present and given an opportunity to express their distress, the parental fighting would have continued even longer and joint custody might never have been negotiated.

As treatment progressed, the chaos and "booms" of earlier pictures gave way to drawings like those in Drawings 6.8 and 6.9. Once again the house motif is uppermost, but now a different feeling is conveyed.

Several sessions after Eric drew Drawings 6.6 and 6.7, he drew a picture of a house and two trees (Drawing 6.8). This drawing contrasts markedly with the earlier house scene (Drawing 6.6), where both his wishes and his denial were more operative. Although the scene depicted here is more serene, the emptiness is profound, and the separation of the two trees symbolizing his two separated parents is notable. About the same time, Jenny also drew her version of a house (Drawing 6.9). Jejuneness is its dominant feature. The house is big, but there are no people, or even curtains, to signify that anyone lives there. Unlike Jenny's earlier pictures (Drawings 6.1 and 6.3), there are no flowers or grass, or color of any kind. Drawings 6.8 and 6.9 accurately

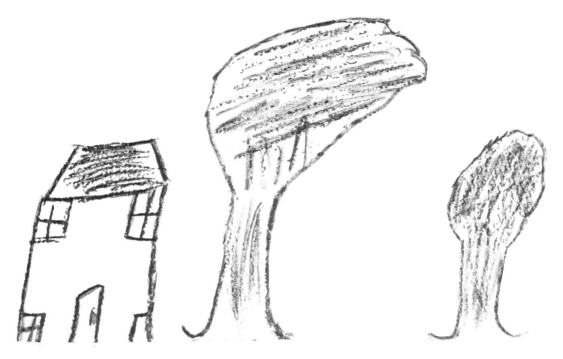

Drawing 6.8

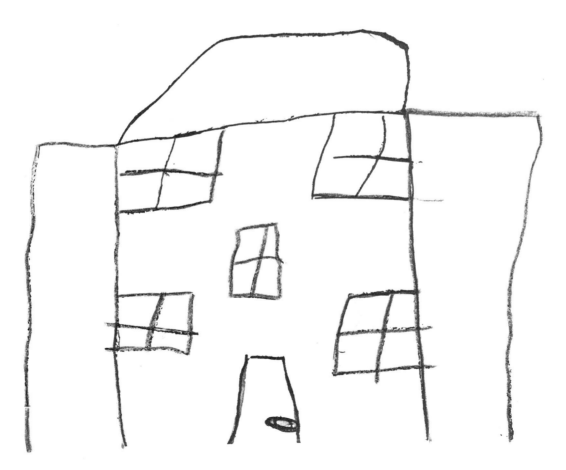

Drawing 6.9

depicted a stage of family treatment. Both children feared they would be abandoned, and the children and their mother experienced a growing feeling of emptiness. The parents argued less; Mrs. Roberts became very thin and cried frequently, and the children worried about their future, since their split family was becoming a reality to them.

Another family reality to be addressed was the need to mourn the passing of family traditions and to establish new patterns befitting a separated family. These emotionally charged issues are always difficult for family members to broach, and the children were often helpful. As the Christmas season drew near, the therapists were struck by the lack of discussion regarding arrangements that would need to be made for the children.

Finally, about two weeks before Christmas, Eric, pointedly and concretely reminded the family with a drawing (Drawing 6.10) that the holiday was near! Eric drew this picture in total silence. When he finished, he handed the drawing directly to one of the therapists, who wondered aloud how the family planned to spend Christmas this year. The therapist, with picture in hand, continued the discussion, pointing to the two sides represented in the picture and commenting that it would be different to have Christmas in two houses. Mrs. Roberts was also upset about the prospect of her first Christmas alone with the children, but she was afraid to initiate a conversation about her husband's plans. Eric's picture provided the opening for a discussion of this topic.

The therapist noted the perfect symmetry of Eric's Christmas drawing. The two sides of the tree hold an exactly equal number of gifts, signifying once again the family split. There are four objects on each side, two red and two black, and outside the tree on each side one red and one black object. Eric's concern about giving to his parents equally, together with his wish to continue to be close to both of them, were clear as well. Once the Christmas holiday had been brought up by Eric's drawing, his parents acknowledged that it would be a difficult time for them also. The family not only was able to discuss plans for the coming holiday, but even agreed on a general arrangement for future years. The children then felt reassured that they would continue to have contact with both parents – now and in the future.

During this middle phase of treatment the drawings made by the children during therapy sessions were more regressed. As the children became more upset their drawings appeared more like the drawings of younger children. Pictures such as Drawings 6.5, 6.6, and 6.7, depicted how overwhelmed and confused the children felt. Like many children whose parents are in heated

104

Drawing 6.10

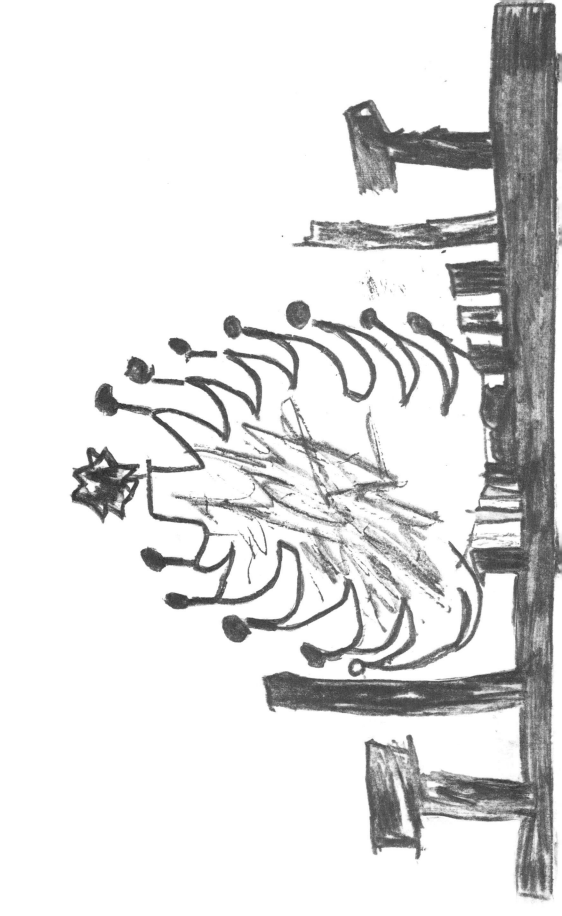

conflict, Eric and Jenny found it difficult to separate themselves from their parents' interactions. At times they felt angry at, torn between, too close to, or overidentified with one parent or the other. However, in Drawing 6.11, Eric drew us a clue that some of the necessary definition and separation from his parents' conflicts had begun to take place. Drawing 6.11 still contains aggressive, emotional clashes of objects in space. The circle and the triangle are mixed vivid orange, red, green, and black. As in many previous instances, Eric drew grass and a tree. However, in contrast to Drawing 6.6, this tree is not being bombarded or split in two, rather it appears sturdy and intact and is made with strong strokes. It is clearly set well into the ground. Significantly, the crashing and clashing occurs somewhat at a distance, permitting other elements of the picture to flourish!

Although the parents continued to disagree in therapy meetings, the family now reported, when questioned, fewer uncontrolled arguments outside the sessions. It appeared that the fighting had become more confined within the boundaries and the relative safety of the therapy hours.

THE CHILDREN'S VIEW OF THE MARITAL AND CHILD-PARENT RELATIONSHIP

Throughout the family treatment both children showed how they felt about themselves and their parents in clear pictures of the relationships among the family members.

As discussed in the previous section, the children frequently were distressed and frightened by the hostility they perceived in their parents' relationship with each other. Perhaps the most poignant of Eric's drawings regarding his parents' battles was his "War Between the Italians and the Americans" (his parents' nationalities by birth!). This was the name he put on this picture (Drawing 6.12) and he identified the sides. Eric drew the opposing armies firing missiles from machine guns directly at each other (the lines go directly from one to the other); he even depicted a dead soldier in the upper left-hand corner of the page. There are differences between the two sides: on the left side the guns are blacker and the figures clearly rounder. On the right side the figures are stick figures with thin guns.

The parents' fights were frightening for the children, who could not be sure that everyone was going to survive. The mother's side contains the dead soldier! Eric drew Drawing 6.12 when his parents were having a heated conversation concerning temporary visitation arrangements. While the argument went on, Eric finished his drawing and gave it to his father. The therapists

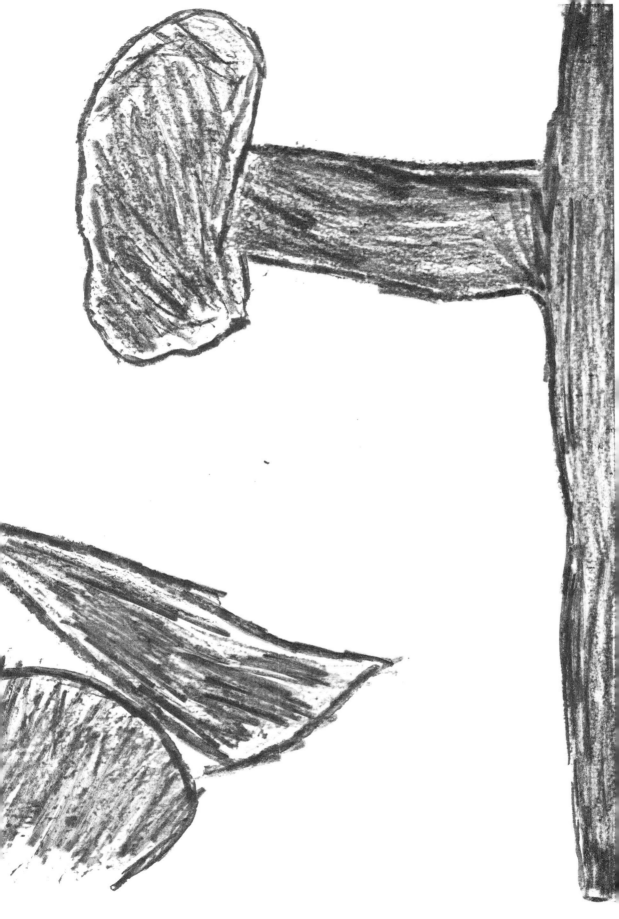

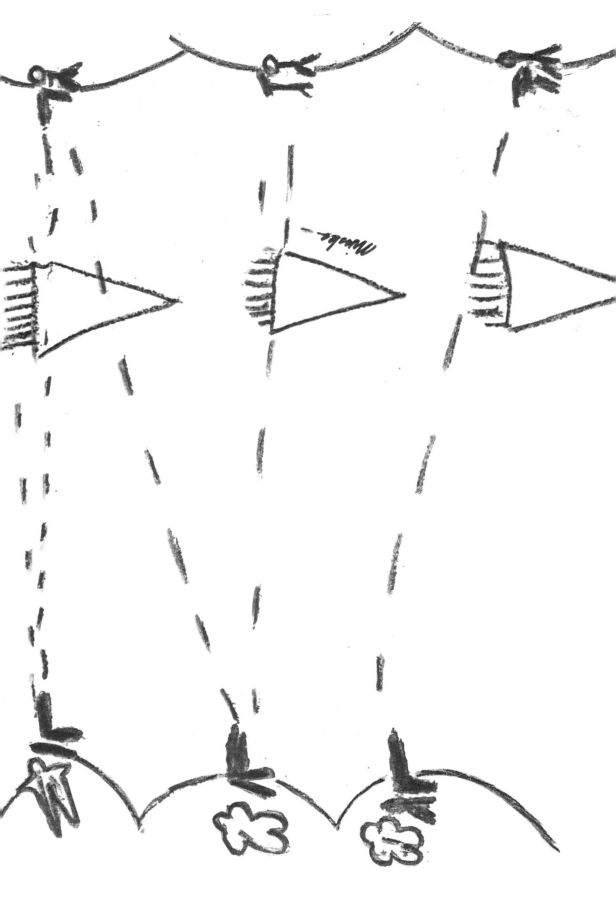

interrupted the parental argument and asked Eric to tell his father about his picture. When the parents learned the name of the picture, "War Between the Italians and the Americans," they laughed, immediately identified the sides, and continued their discussion under better control.

Along with drawing in sessions, the children also made up plays separately and together, using each other as participants, or occasionally enlisting some of the adults as characters in these plays. At times, after quietly rehearsing under a table, they emerged and put on a play in the open, specifically for the adults. "Playing house" together was another favorite game. Frequently, they pretended with their dolls or puppets to be a "happy" family doing many things together. For example, the "husband and wife" dolls would take their babies out in the carriage for a walk. The meaning of these wishful themes was so obvious to the parents that this play afforded frequent opportunities for the family to reminisce and talk together about how sad a divorce was for everyone.

Play, like the drawings, served various functions. The content of the children's play sequences often alerted the therapists to then current family difficulties. For example, in two consecutive sessions the children played a game they invented called "Bus." This game used all the people and much of the furniture in the therapy room. The children took all the chairs in the therapy room and lined them up, one behind another, so that the room was divided in half, and placed one parent at each side of the room. They asked the female therapist to be the bus driver and they gave her a schedule of stops. The "bus" made many stops and had frequent, serious misadventures. Often Eric and Jenny would miss the bus, or the bus would pass them by, leaving them stranded and miserable.

The therapists were somewhat uncertain of the full meaning of this rather complicated and repeated game, although some feelings and issues were apparent. The children seemed to be trying to communicate something more specific and important. When asked about these "play" bus trips, it was learned that the children had, in fact, recently begun to take public transportation from one parent's home to the other. The parents had numerous quarrels about the excessive traveling time required by the visitation schedule. They hinted at their thoughts that they wanted the children to begin to travel a little on their own. The children confessed that they worried that their parents would not meet them at their stop and they would be alone and lost. Such abandonment fears are frequent in the course of a divorce. Both parents were then able to reassure the children that, even though there were fights and disagreements, they would be met reliably and never asked to travel when they felt too frightened.

Drawing 6.12

Although the children were often preoccupied with their parents' difficult relationship, which became the subject of many of their drawings, they also depicted their ideas about their own relationships with their parents.

At times during the treatment, Eric became the object of his parents' concern, and even of their disappointment. In one particular session, Mr. Roberts complained about his son's lack of athletic ability, his marginal school performance, and his encopresis. Mrs. Roberts, who often took her son's side, remained silent, listening to her husband's criticisms. Although the father asked his son for explanations for his behavior, Eric sat quietly. The therapist then asked the parents for more details in order to better understand the parents' complaints. While the adults spoke, Eric retreated to the playtable and drew. This time, however, he did not offer to show the therapists or his parents the drawing, and only hesitantly showed it upon request. The picture (Drawing 6.13) shows a large green bird hovering over and yelling at a smaller brown bird. The green bird has a large, dark beak and is yelling "DUM, DUM, DUM." The smaller bird, who has no noticeable beak, replies in shaky letters, "I'm slow," and "BABY." When we ask Eric about this, he told us the little chicken was so frightened that he was shaking; and it appeared to us that Eric was feeling shaken in this session as well.

Although Eric was hesitant to show his father this drawing, the therapists encouraged him to do so. Once the father recognized how his criticisms affected his son, he became more patient and sought ways to be helpful. We encouraged Mr. Roberts in these efforts, for example, to practice throwing and catching a baseball with Eric before Eric's Little League games (Note 2).

Later in treatment, Eric drew another picture of himself and his father (Drawing 6.14). The two figures are inside an igloo, cold and insulated in their protective suits, and are throwing logs into a stove trying to keep warm. Here the larger figure is no longer derogating the smaller one and they seem to be able to act peaceably together. But Eric showed us in this picture that he still felt isolated from his father and needed to protect himself from his father's past and/or potential criticism.

Eric and his mother were very close and he was often worried about her. In Drawing 6.15 Eric drew a "flower lady" with a sad, red mouth saying "Hi." It is striking that, although this lady was saying "Hi," she was not doing "Hi," that is, he portrayed her frowning, without hands, and unable to reach out. Eric was capable of drawing hands but had not, so the therapists understood the emotional significance of the "flower lady." During this time in treatment Mrs. Roberts seemed barely overtly angry, but Eric recognized and conveyed her depression at a time when she could not.

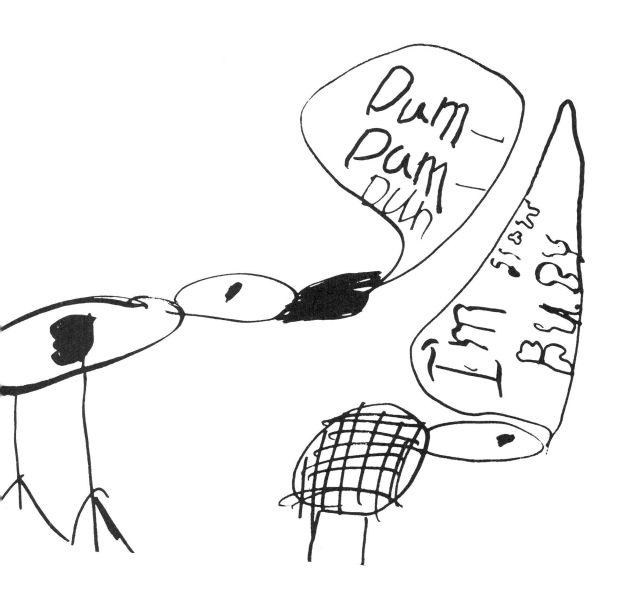

Drawing 6.13

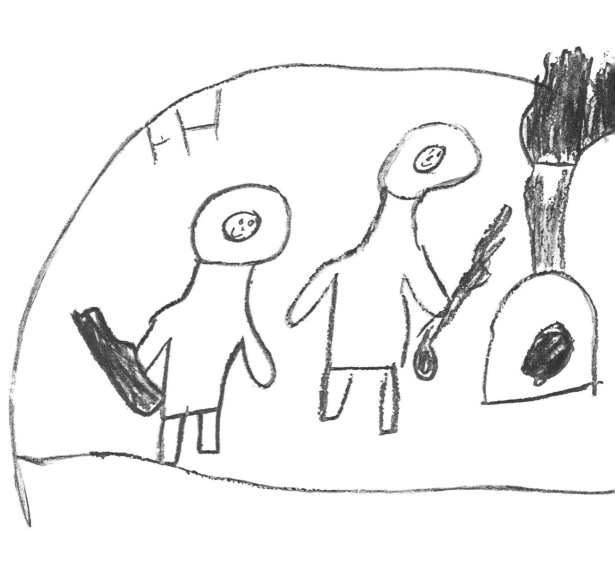

Drawing 6.14

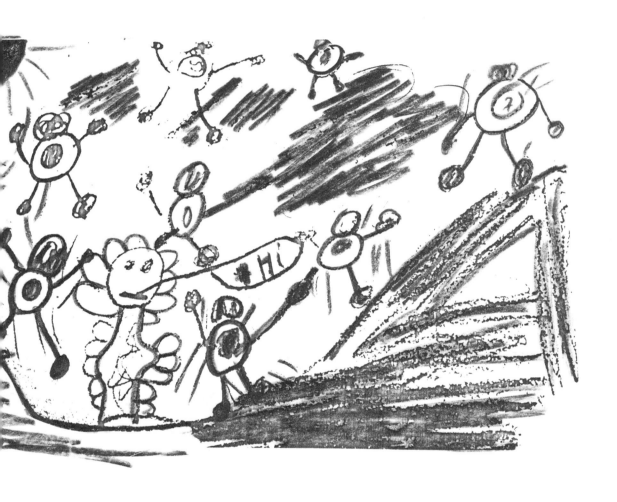

Drawing 6.15

Drawing 6.15 depicts the sad "flower lady" surrounded by chaos, besieged by eight purple spacemen running down a hill and descending from the sky toward her. Eric used these space creatures to represent himself with his mother. But, unlike the situation with many other pictures, which Eric would explain and talk about, when asked what was happening in this picture, he merely shrugged his shoulders and turned his attention to another activity. Eric expressed concern about his mother in this picture, but could not speak directly about it when others, particularly his mother, had not yet been able to identify and address her depressed feelings.

THE CHILDREN'S MESSAGES ABOUT THEMSELVES

As the parents' feelings and decisions about their lives and their divorce changed, the children were deeply affected. The children carefully chronicled these personal, internal changes in their drawings, leaving the pictures behind in the therapy room for the therapists to keep. While in the previous sections the focus was on the children's representations of familial themes and relationships, the following drawings depict the children's feelings about themselves.

Jenny

As previously mentioned, Jenny's role in her family at the outset of treatment was to be happy, expressive, and competent, never sad or tearful. In Drawing 6.16 she characteristically represents herself as a large red and yellow flower. The flower blooms under a blue sky and bright yellow sun and is placed close to a tree. The flower and the tree are huddled together in the corner of the page. When she completed it, Jenny handed this picture directly to her mother. The tree represents her mother and Jenny places herself, the flower, close by. This drawing, and many similar ones, represented Jenny's effort to be cheerful and giving for the sake of her upset parent.

Early in treatment, Jenny drew a self-portrait (Drawing 6.17) and showed it to the family. Again she used bright, cheerful colors. She is wearing a "party dress," her arms are swinging, and she mouths a happy "Hi." She identified the girl clearly by labeling it "me." Although her life had been uprooted and her parents, at this time, were fighting, she presented herself as a happy child. It was only after several months of treatment that she revealed herself to be just the opposite.

Shortly before Easter vacation, Jenny drew a multicolored Easter egg which had fallen off a bridge into black water (Drawing 6.18). The emotional

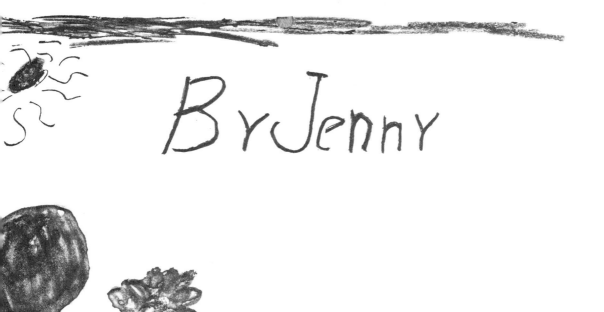

By Jenny

Drawing 6.16

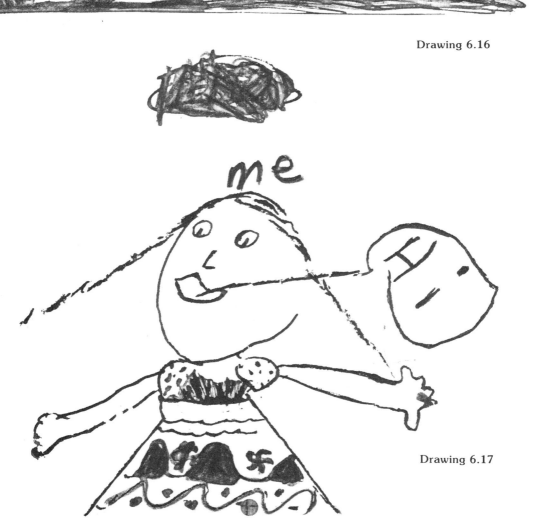

me

Drawing 6.17

text of this picture appears similar to that of her brother's drawing (Drawing 6.6) in which he concretely labeled the images and drew arrows for emphasis. Explaining her drawing, Jenny told a story about a silly Easter egg who, while walking on the bridge, fell into the water. The colors on this Easter egg are the same as the colors of Jenny's flowers. This time, however, there is no sun or blue sky and the bright colors (hot pink, yellow, and orange) are surrounded by black. This is an apt depiction of her dilemma of trying to be happy and pretty in the midst of black anger, depression, and chaos.

Shortly after Easter, Jenny began to draw her unhappiness in a less disguised way. In Drawing 6.19 there are early signs of anger and self-derogation. Jenny wrote "this is Jenny" on the picture but draws her body chopped in half and prints "BAD" next to her self-portrait. She evidently intended, at first, to give this picture to her mother, but she changed her mind and crossed out the dedication. This drawing with its crossing-out and with a "mistake" in the upper left-hand corner is unusual for Jenny and appears less organized than her previous work.

In Drawing 6.20 her drawing and self-portrayal became even more sloppy and regressed. Although she began with bright colors, she crayoned over these with a heavy layer of black, so that hints of brightness show through only slightly. She poignantly writes her name over the picture and labels it

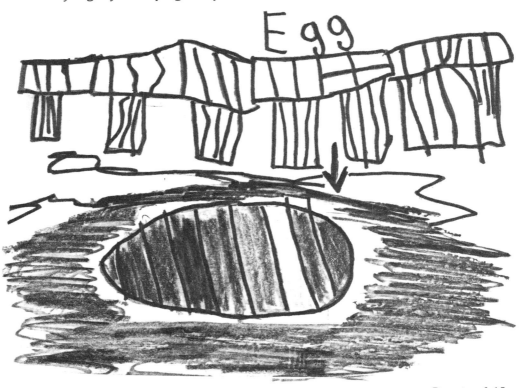

Drawing 6.18

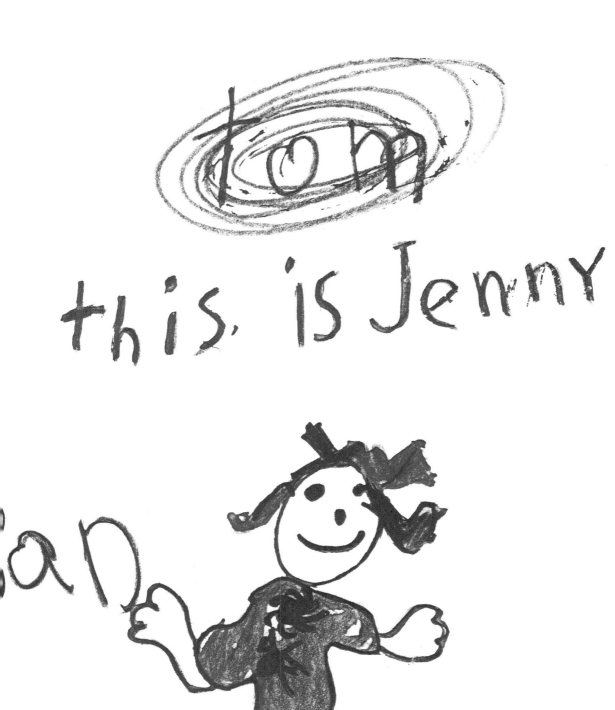

Drawing 6.19

"A weird design." This is the least organized drawing Jenny ever made; it communicates her shame and despair. Jenny was showing her upset, and the therapists actively used her drawings to help her tell her parents how she felt. They commented on how long it had been since Jenny drew pretty flowers or pictures of herself playing and smiling, and said they thought she was sad. The parents wanted at least one of their children to be "happy and problem-free," and had, therefore, denied Jenny's unhappiness for a long time. As this discussion ensued, Jenny drew a big, teary-eyed, sad face (Drawing 6.21), as if to confirm the therapists' comments and interpretation. Her mother added that Jenny did seem upset at home and that Jenny complained loudly about the living arrangements when she visited her father. Both parents acknowledged that their usually strong daughter needed some special consideration during this difficult time.

Near the end of treatment Jenny drew a portrait that combined her features with those of the female co-therapist (Drawing 6.22). The dark hair and earrings of the therapist were combined with Jenny's blue eyes, long hair, ribbons, and freckles. She no longer pretended to be a happy flower. Her family had divorced, her father wanted to remarry, and her mother was still unhappy. Furthermore, therapy was ending and she had grown fond of the therapists, who knew Jenny and her family well.

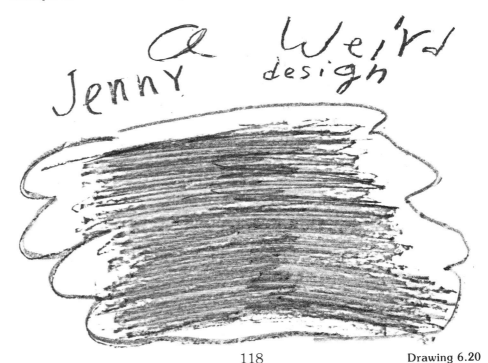

118 **Drawing 6.20**

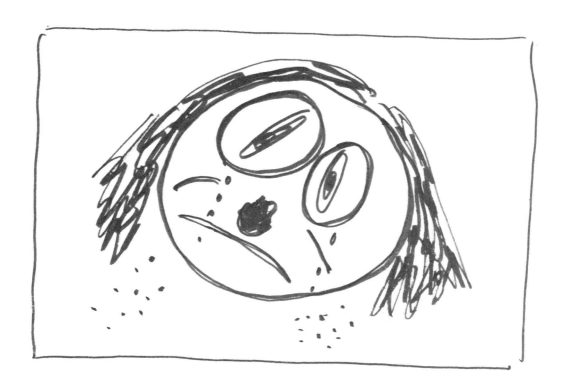

Drawing 6.21

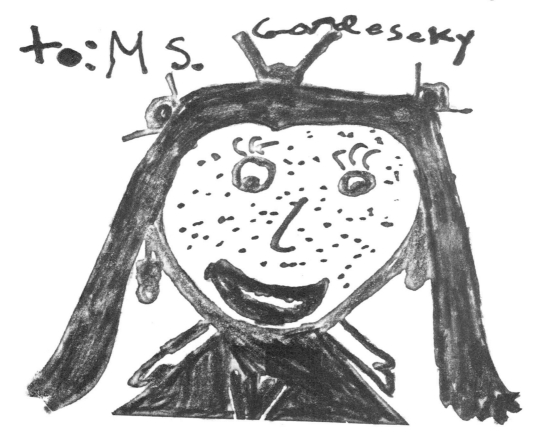

Drawing 6.22

Eric

Although Mr. Roberts initially sought family therapy to help with the impending planned divorce, almost immediately Eric was revealed as a boy with his own problems. As stated previously, Eric was encopretic and performed well below his intellectual potential in school. Throughout treatment both parents seemed to worry more about Eric than about Jenny.

From the beginning, Eric's drawings were filled with strong marks of both fear and aggression. In Drawing 6.23 he depicts both of these aspects of his inner experiences. He creates a huge brown monster with evil eyes and sharp, jagged teeth. There is a war raging and the monster is being attacked from the ground and the air by guns and green military fighter planes. The houses are on fire as the monster makes his path through the destruction. Small figures crying for help are being flung aside as the monster captures in his palm another crying figure saying "ouch." This picture dramatically revealed Eric's fears of being attacked and overwhelmed, while simultaneously expressing his own aggressive, omnipotent fantasies.

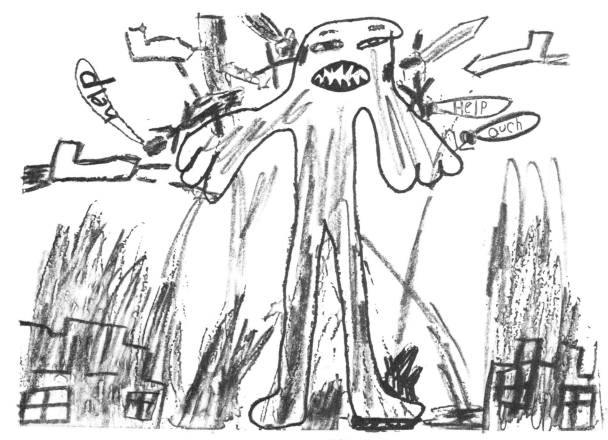

Drawing 6.23

Eric's self-esteem suffered. His portrait of a "freckle-faced freak" was drawn three months into treatment (Drawing 6.24). This picture clearly portrays his profoundly distorted self-image and his devalued feelings about himself. He draws himself without a body and with his eyes and nose barely sketched in. Thus, when Eric did not feel overwhelmed with anxiety and anger, this was what remained. Eric's drawings told the therapists about his neediness, and they helped the parents recognize their son's need to become competent and valued, regardless of their own unresolved issues. For example, Eric's need to have friends his own age to play with was discussed as something that the parents needed to plan for together, if Eric was to spend time with each of them on the weekends.

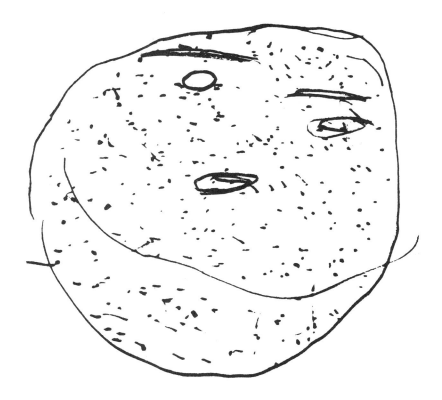

Drawing 6.24

121

Much later in treatment, Eric gave the male co-therapist a portrait of "Bozo the Clown" (Drawing 6.25). As in Drawing 6.24, only a head is drawn, although this picture is more organized and contains more detail and color than the earlier drawing. Eric gives Bozo a red nose, mouth, and cheeks, blue eyes, and two big ears. Perhaps the large ears signify that both Eric and the therapist listened carefully over the past year. Eric's self-image had changed during that year from a destructive, fearful monster, to a devalued freak, and finally to a clown. In fact, Eric was more lively in therapy sessions and demonstrated his clever sense of humor in the plays he and his sister performed. Eric asked to join a drama class and each parent agreed to drive him to class on alternative weeks.

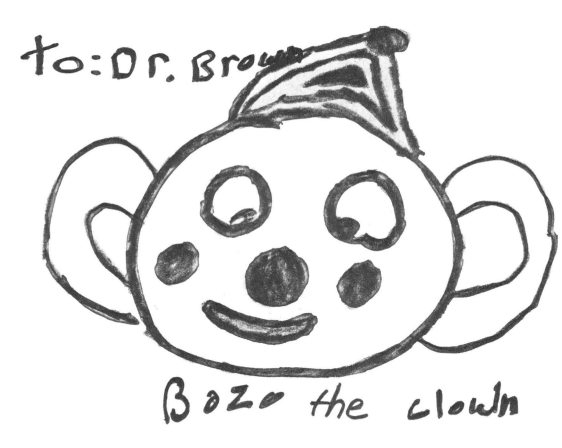

Drawing 6.25

SUMMARY

Eric and Jenny's play and drawings introduced, clarified, and deepened the therapists' understanding of the Roberts family. Throughout the family treatment, the children vividly illustrated how they felt about themselves, their parents, and their family's separation.

The family was in treatment for 15 months during which time there were many difficult periods when both the family and the therapists felt frustrated. Because the parents were often so angry and appeared to be working at such serious cross-purposes, the therapists were occasionally tempted to treat them only as a couple and thus "protect" the children from more arguments. Also, when the children so dramatically depicted their internalized conflicts and anger, the therapists thought of referring each of them for individual therapy. But, throughout, and in retrospect, it seemed that either format would have yielded an incomplete "picture," and perhaps an incomplete result. For example, it was only when the children graphically demonstrated their pain, anger, and confusion, that their parents could set aside their disappointment with each other and focus on their children's needs. Furthermore, despite the parents' disagreements, they continued to trust that their children would benefit from having a stable relationship with both of them. It made sense for this family, at this time, to resolve their difficulties together rather than separately.

FOLLOW-UP

Many years have passed since the Roberts' family treatment period took place. The therapists contacted both parents and invited them and their children to meet to talk about publishing their family story, including some pictures the children had drawn in therapy sessions. Mr. Roberts had remarried and he and his new wife and baby moved into the same community where his children and their mother lived. Both Eric and Jenny were frequent visitors at their father's new house and reportedly enjoyed their new half-brother. Mrs. Roberts looked back at the earlier time of the separation and divorce as very difficult, but now has a congenial relationship with Mr. Roberts. She is glad that the children have access to the rest of their family and she feels that the children are doing well.

CHAPTER NOTES

1) These categories are not all-inclusive. They do not encompass the full range of children's drawings that occur in the course of family treatment.
2) We previously commented on the one-sided encouragement of fathers to play more with their sons. In this intervention we inadvertently repeated the same lop-sided practice we mentioned previously – mother and daughter were neither mentioned nor encouraged!

7

How-To: Some Specifics on Young Children in Family Therapy

HOW-TO

Why another discussion of "how-to" in family therapy, when the field already has so many schools, each with its own techniques, strategies, prescriptions, and other technical advances? These are offered because they focus particularly on children in family therapy who require special, concrete attention. The descriptions will not fit exactly any particular family therapy school or style. They are a mixture that has developed in the course of years of clinical practice.

What is a how-to? It is like a recipe for chicken soup or chocolate chip cookies. The regional variations of those recipes, though tasting quite different, can all be used to treat whatever ails you! Our brand is New England, with a heavy sprinkling of developmental psychoanalytic spices.

Since this chapter is on how-to, the language is often like recipe language: make, do, and add. These expressions emphasize specifics but should

be read only as an opinion and a recommendation. Personal style and therapist preference are also necessary ingredients of a family therapy recipe. So,
although parts of this chapter may sound like injunctions, read them primarily
as description rather than prescription and, for yourselves as family therapists
including young children, season with an ounce, or preferably many ounces,
of self-expression!

This chapter will cover:

1) Introductions: Saying "Hello" to Children;
2) Supplies: Equipment for Children;
3) Parents' Reactions to Supplies–Play Materials;
4) Messes Children Make;
5) Going to the Bathroom: Bathroom Play;
6) Pictures: Look, See, Feel; and
7) Celebrations: Birthdays, Holidays, and Other Special Occasions.

Photographic sequences will illustrate these how-to's. They are additional
separate examples, not illustrations of the case vignettes in the text.

INTRODUCTIONS: SAYING "HELLO" TO CHILDREN

Hello! The therapist's first greeting to a family brings into immediate focus
the special attention needed by young children. It is easy to overlook the
little ones who are gathered below your knee. After, or perhaps even before,
greeting the adults, usually by a handshake, bend down to the child's eye
level! This is not the usual behavior of polite adult society, where to include
children in a greeting, adults usually lean over them.

Though your knees may creak, try to achieve actual, level, eye contact
with the young children. Adult-oriented therapists may automatically extend
their hand in greeting to a child as to an adult. Watch carefully because the
children may be too frightened for hand touching – or any touching – but eye
contact cannot hurt. Your adult bones and joints are no excuse! In the same
way, babies may be recognized with a gentle touch and a look. It must all
be soft and low-keyed. It is most important not to overlook any member of
the family in this first greeting. If the family is large and active, and its members,
particularly the children, immediately move about, you may have to ask, "Have
I missed anyone?" Then a little voice may be heard or a small child may point
out their overlooked sibling, either older or younger. Babies may want to touch
you as their form of greeting. The therapist must be ready to receive "hello"
in many forms:

126

"I couldn't leave her home. I have nobody – but she smells." Mother paused momentarily and added, "Hello. I am Mrs. Jones and this is Jeannie." Mr. Jones came from somewhere behind as the therapist returned the greetings and included Mr. Jones. Mrs. Jones led the way into the office holding the odoriferous baby at arm's length. Jeannie, the baby, put her hands out toward the therapist's brightly colored, shiny beads. That was her hello! The therapist returned the greeting, putting her arms out for the baby, and simultaneously asked whether Mrs. Jones wanted to change the baby on the nearby couch. The therapist was quite aware of not wanting to hold Jeannie for long, but she did want to acknowledge the baby's first greeting in family therapy.

This example of a hello how-to may seem simple and obvious. But, it is so easy to leave out babies or the young, nonverbal members of the family because they are not yet of "speaking-hello" age. But they can touch, look, and smell "hello." It is likely they will know if they are left out, although they do not yet speak out directly, in adult words.

After the therapist has invited the family into the office, and exchanged a few pleasantries, another specific introductory point arises that is most important to young children. The therapist must find out in a general way, but rather quickly, what the young children have been told about coming to the session. Many abstruse, euphemistic, and strange things are told to children, and the sooner these are brought into the open and discussed, the better:

After the first few minutes of settling in, John, age five, kept moving his head and eyes pronouncedly up, down, and around, from the therapist to the playtable and then up again all along the ceiling. The head movements were so marked that the therapist asked what he was looking for. John answered, "Where are the lollipops and balloons?" He had been told that he was coming to visit a place with balloons and lollipops.

In another family's first session, a younger child, age three, after the initial family introductory noise decreased, repeatedly said, "When are we getting on the bus ride?" This seemed odd until the therapist asked, "What have the children been told about coming to this family session?" This was a suburban family coming to an urban clinic. In making the rather complicated arrangements for the whole family to be at the session, there was a brief time when it seemed that part of the family, Mother and three-year-old, would

I. INTRODUCTIONS: SAYING "HELLO" TO CHILDREN

The children, Kenny, age two and Jane, age five, preceded the parents into the office. Jane had already made herself comfortable in the waiting room by taking her shoes off. The younger sibling, Kenny, grabbed the toy telephone and started to "talk." Prior to this first session, he was told that he was coming to a "talking lady," and he was ready! Still at the door, the therapist greets the parents while Jane notices Sock-o. (Photo 7.1)

Jane brings her brother's attention to her business and away from his "talk" on the telephone. The therapist crouches down and says hello to the children. (Photo 7.2)

Moving further into the office, the therapist again crouches to greet Kenny and Jane. Kenny and the therapist meet eye-to-eye, as Jane looks to her parents, who tell her to say hello. (Photo 7.3)

Kenny moves back, no touch or handshake allowed, and the therapist keeps her place unchanged as Jane tells her her name. Notice that Father (only chest and body seen within picture) has moved farther into the room. Mother, holding back, cannot be seen in this picture. (Photo 7.4)

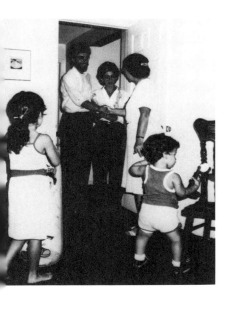

Photo 7.1

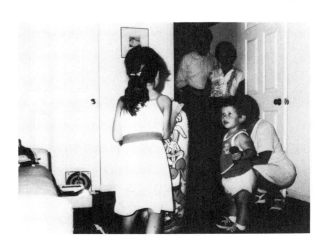

Photo 7.2

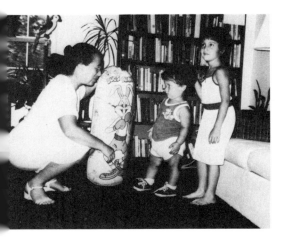

Photo 7.3

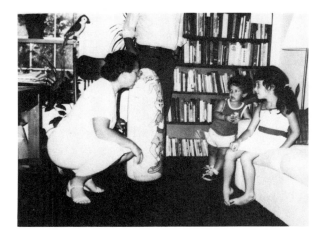

Photo 7.4

129

have to take the bus rather than ride in their old station wagon. But they had all come together in the station wagon. This "bus ride" idea was exciting for the three-year-old, and he was impatient for the real fun – the bus ride – to begin!

What the children are told about coming to the family session leads to the next topic: "What are we here to do?"

The discussion should be kept very simple, using few and little words. We do not expect children to understand the complexities of "problems," but rather that the family is coming all together to talk about many things, including their "troubles:"

> John was not told that the family therapy session was not a place for lollipops and balloons. The therapist asked what kind of candy and balloons he liked. John was told that the therapist liked to know the special "likes" of John and of all of the other family members. This discussion of "likes" then turned to "dislikes," which was followed by an explanation about being here to find out and talk about the family likes, dislikes, troubles, and many other things.

> In the opening session with the suburban family, the "fun" of a bus ride was directly acknowledged, not contradicted, as the specifics of transportation to the session were discussed. The therapist then led the discussion from "fun" to other potential contents of family discussions in therapy sessions. The discussion of fun added a positive note to talk about troubles in the family. The bus ride became an asset rather than an incorrect explanation or mistake.

It is important to make a simple explanation of the purposes of the session. After hearing the explanations that have been given to the children, this should be done without contradicting what may have been said by parents and siblings. Instead, the therapist should gently substitute an explanation that will begin the process of creating a safe and therapeutic environment.

As the therapist makes introductory contact with all members of the family, the parents may push the introductions toward an immediate focus on the "identified" or symptomatic child. While it may be necessary to recognize this special status, the therapist should not allow this recognition to interfere with direct acknowledgement of all members of the family. Other simple ways of making contact, in addition to eye contact, are brief comments about clothing, which is particularly appropriate for teens. Any item, a doll, toy, book, tie, or other special piece of clothing, that has been brought by any member of the family warrants a simple, brief comment. The purpose of including everyone and their things is to begin the process of making every family member comfortable within this new and strange setting.

Another brief contact with each member of the family toward the end is a useful way to finish the session. By then some children may be less frightened, so that the end contact might be a little touch or good-bye. Again, it is important that there be some kind of contact with each member of the family. No one is omitted or excluded because of age or any other characteristic.

SUPPLIES: EQUIPMENT FOR CHILDREN

What kinds of toys does a therapist need in order to include children in a family session? The answer is simple. How nice that in one area of practice there is a simple answer! But first, an explanation and a question.

There is a "developmental line" (A. Freud, 1981a), which has been described in an earlier chapter on play (Note 1), that occurs as children progress in their growth and development from play to work: from enjoying simple toys, handling a rattle, or looking at a hanging mobile to using complicated construction sets. Is a representative toy from each stage of development necessary for equipping the family therapy room? Recognizing the need for children to play, and knowing something about child development, may make it seem that supplying the office will become a very complex job. However, the paramount purpose of supplies is quite different from encompassing child development. As discussed in Chapter 2, play materials promote easy child-level expression and provide an outlet for nonverbal reduction of anxiety and diversion when necessary. Thus, simple materials – paper, magic markers, crayons, play-dough, a few toys, a baby doll, a family of small dolls (mother, father, children), a bowl of candy, like M&M's, or simple food, like nuts or raisins – are really quite sufficient. These few toys can be used in many diverse ways:

When a session to include the entire L family was discussed, the family complained about bringing the youngest child, Anne, age seven, because, they said, "She cannot sit still." The parents had not brought her to previous sessions because they were concerned that her active behavior would be "too much" in the office. In this case, it had not been established initially by the therapists

131

II. SUPPLIES: EQUIPMENT FOR CHILDREN

1) Jane lets her fist go at the Sock-o as Kenny watches. (Photo 7.5)

She teaches Kenny how to hit this toy. Notice Mother's worried expression and the therapist's delight! (Photo 7.6)

2) M&M's make an interesting face. This one is sad. Kenny and his parents watch intently. Kenny looks sad also. (Photo 7.7)

But the face was not sad enough, and Jane fixes the M&M mouth with her mouth to accentuate the feeling. (Photo 7.8)

Jane adds a body around the face. Her little brother wants to help, but is told "Don't touch!" by Mother. (Photo 7.9)

Jane eats the last piece of this person. Kenny finally joins his sister in eating the extras in the bowl. Father is pleased with Kenny; Mother backs off. (Photo 7.10)

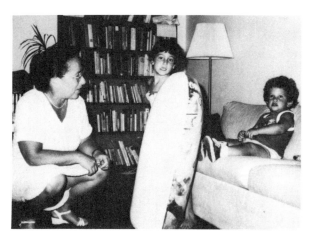
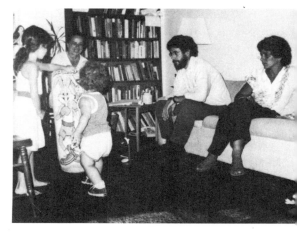

Photo 7.5

Photo 7.

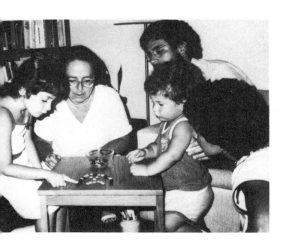

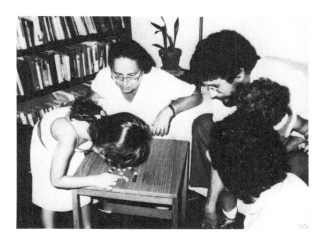

Photo 7.7

Photo 7.8

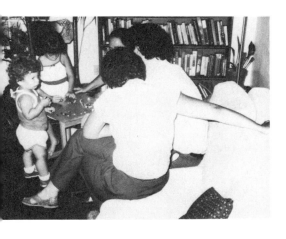

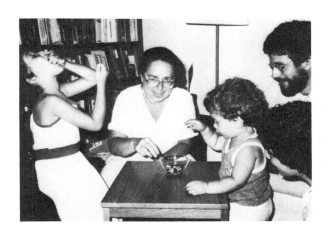

Photo 7.9

Photo 7.10

that it was important at this time to meet the entire family. This was explained and the child was brought to the next session. The therapists put only paper, crayons, M&M's, and a small doll on a low table (Note 2). After eye-level introductions, the session began with a quick question from Anne. The seven-year-old immediately asked about using the materials and was given the simple permission by the therapist, "The materials are there for anybody to use." This explanation was enlarged and strengthened by "going around" via contact between the therapists and all family members, including the adults. Anne carefully opened the M&M packet and made the outline of a person, specifically choosing only the brown M&M's. She saved the few brightly colored candies for the last touches. These, two red eyes, a yellow nose, and three green ones as the mouth, became the features of the face.

Family members continued their heated conversation as the seven-year-old slowly, while quietly sitting in one place, ate the person piece by piece. This contented cannibalism ended just a few minutes before the end of the hour. As she finished the last M&M, Anne beamed at the therapist and said, "That was yummy!" The therapist agreed! Clearly good contact had been made with this "difficult" and active child.

There was a wide age division in this family. The next older child was a late adolescent who had argued heatedly with the parents throughout the entire session. In this particular session it would have been futile to attempt any lengthy or verbal inclusion of the youngest child. But play inclusion was easy, expressive, and fun!

There is always room for both personal preferences in and objections to supplies, either by therapist or by family member. Rarely does anyone object to paper, crayons, or clay. Some people do object to candy. If such a statement is loudly voiced by a family member, it is easy to put the bowl away, since the intent is to provide an alternative, child-appropriate avenue of expression to talk.

Board games seem to us not useful in family therapy sessions. These games such as Monopoly are too long, too complicated, and not easily manipulable by the therapist. In addition, in terms of outcome, i.e., winning or losing, there is usually a good deal of luck, as well as skill, involved in playing these games, which is very distracting for the therapist. If, however, a child brings in a favorite board game or other toy, it should be received appropriately, and with pleasure, and included in some fashion in the day's session.

Some favorite toys may seem to be impediments to talk, but the therapist must manage to include and cherish them in the session in a noninterfering way:

> Paul, a two-year-old, entered the family therapy room carrying his favorite toy, a jack-in-the-box. "Jack" clattered and made a lot of noise as Paul began to enthusiastically play with it. The mother stated that this was the toy that the child loved the most, was rarely separated from, and that Paul had insisted on bringing it to the session. The therapist admired "Jack" loudly and asked if he could hold it so that he could see the colors better. Paul was pleased, brought it over, and actually handed the clattering toy to the therapist. This maneuver reduced the noise – the many colors to admire closely and feel quietly kept "Jack" in the hands of the therapist for a considerable portion of the session.

Since one maneuver does not always work, several different strategies may have to be devised. Playfulness and imagination on the part of the therapist will aid such attempts. A particular kind of toy may be introduced for a specific purpose. For example, the nonverbal, playful release of aggression is facilitated by having an object that is designated for hitting. This can be a large, indestructible pillow or a more defined punching toy, such as a plastic "Sock-o" which moves from side to side ringing as it is punched.

Some toys can be brought out quite deliberately in later sessions, when the therapeutic need becomes clear. Safety and limits within the room should have been discussed previously, elaborated on, and tested in earlier sessions. The therapist can take away a toy or other play material between sessions when, in the course of several sessions, it has provided mostly interference and nonuseful expression:

> Billy produced finger paintings one after another, in very large quantity, handing them to parents, therapists, and covering every available space for them to dry. Neediness was discussed, limits set, and distraction from difficult talk became an issue. Nevertheless, the finger paintings, an unabated "snow job," continued. The therapists felt stymied. Much to the therapists' surprise, the supervisor suggested, "Take away the finger paints and paper before the next session." In the next session, when Billy discovered that there

135

was no paint or paper, he was startled and became very angry. His parents looked terrified and made no comment. That particular session and subsequent ones continued without the paints and paper. The parents' fear of this child's anger and their inability to set limits now became available therapeutic issues.

PARENTS' REACTIONS TO SUPPLIES—PLAY MATERIALS

Inevitably, the presence of play materials, crayons, paper, food, and other supplies is noticed by all family members. Some parents make no overt comments, while others ask, "What about us?" This reaction is delightful and easy to answer by saying, "The materials and supplies are for everyone to use." The therapist should be prepared to supply a considerable amount of paper or play-dough, because it is likely that the supplies will be used in large quantities by family members. When paper or another item runs out, as inevitably occurs, it is most interesting to watch the many kinds of reactions, rivalry, disappointment, or rage that appear.

However, objections to materials are more frequent than use by parents. These objections may not be expressed as direct statements of parental opinion. They may say, "Johnny is not paying attention. He is playing. We are not here for fun." It is likely that this discussion will provide the opportunity for therapeutic entry into problems and aspects of dysfunction in family life. Other objections by parents, such as, "They are too noisy in our session when they play," or, "They are not behaving like good children when they mess with that stuff [play-dough]; they should sit still and be quiet," may also reflect family problems. A simple explanation of the role of play in children's development does not always suffice:

A very "good" boy was referred for serious learning difficulties. As his parents droned on in a boring recital of normal developmental milestones, David, age seven, dressed in a bow tie and long-sleeved shirt, sat motionless in his chair. In the opening minutes of this family interview, the therapist gave the usual explanation of the materials being there for everyone to use. However, it was quite clear that this permission was not sufficient. The parents continued to converse calmly with minimal overt signs of their concerns.

The years prior to the birth of this child had been turbulent and stormy for the family. Violent temper outbursts and aggressive activity outside the family by father led to his lengthy imprisonment.

In his early years, David played for many hours in a prison yard. However, this history was kept secret and David was told that the prison yard was the "grounds of a hospital."

During this interview, the parents spoke euphemistically, in language which indicated to the interviewer that they wished this to continue as a secret. During a pause in the recital of the normal developmental material, the therapist moved his chair over next to the boy and invited him to explore the previously unused play materials. The boy, not looking directly at his parents, asked for their permission, which the interviewer answered with a simple explanation. The parents agreed only after extensive further discussion about permissible and safe activity within this therapy session. The boy then drew a picture of an encased, heavily imprisoned monster, which he said was about to do injury but nobody would be able to see it (like the hidden crimes of violence of his father).

This boy's motor and other "aggressive" play activities had been actively discouraged by both parents, and so were not available for cognitive learning, or other motor and age-appropriate activities. In this instance, the interviewer actively joined with the child after the first permission proved insufficient. Further discussion with the parents about their attitudes toward and fears of activity and play led to the emergence within the family sessions of many problems. The encased monster had multiple meanings, which were not interpreted to the family, but the child's use of his imagination in the picture enabled him to speak. Both Mother and Father feared "badness," and activity and play had become "bad." It was most important to the parents that this boy remain "good" and unknowing. They said, "He has to behave like a good child or else he may grow up wrong." Good children, according to the parents, do not make noise, they sit still, and are otherwise increasingly inhibited in their behavior.

We note that parents are similar to many adult therapists. The parents also may have had previous experience with talking therapies – quiet, contained, with little physical movement occurring within the therapy room. Such experiences may provoke reasonable, nonproblematic questions, e.g., What is this therapy all about? Why not just talk? What is the use of this noise and mess? These questions must be answered specifically, according to the meaning of the particular question. But first, the issue of the use of play material in family therapy must be resolved within the therapist, if s/he is to be available and open to resistance and opposition by parents. (See Chapter 2 for a discussion of this issue for therapists.)

III. PARENTS' REACTIONS TO SUPPLIES - PLAY MATERIALS

Mother is quite concerned with Jane's vigorous and aggressive use of Sock-o. Father is pleased and Kenny pouts because his sister will not let him play. (Photo 7.11)

As Jane pulls the puppets away from Kenny for herself, Mother is again disapproving. (Photo 7.12)

Mother is uncertain about giving the pen in her (Mother's) hand, which Kenny found in the office, back to her son. Kenny, meanwhile, withdraws from the action to draw by himself. (Photo 7.13)

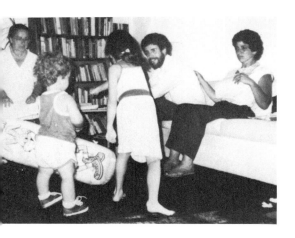

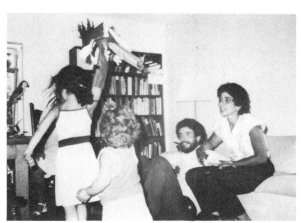

Photo 7.11

Photo 7.12

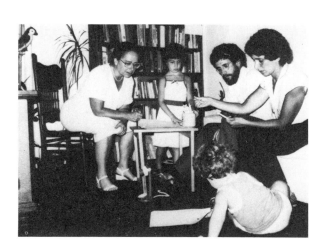

Photo 7.13

139

MESSES CHILDREN MAKE

The messes children make are feared more beforehand than as actual experience. Therapists often imagine large, dirty, and overwhelming messes as they consider the possibility of young children coming to their beautiful, clean offices. But the material of family therapy is not like free association! The experience of encouraging dirty thoughts and "messing around" with words and ideas is quite different from the material of a family therapy session. "No," "Don't," and hands-on control are possible, useful, and will prevent a small mess from developing further. Confusion within the therapist between words and actions may cause excessive fear of messes children might make.

Office space for family therapy that includes children should be kept simple, but should not necessarily be totally child-proof. There is a big difference between daily living at home with small children and a therapy session with small children. At home, children may be out of sight and unsupervised for long periods of time. This obviously is not the case in the office where being out of sight is easily prevented. Very breakable or valuable office objects should be kept out of reach so that children have some freedom or space to move around. Indelible ink and other spillable, stainable, or unwashable materials should not be easily available or possibly not available at all. But beyond these reasonable requirements, the concern about mess is really a fear of young children being present:

> Alice, a toddler, began to scribble on some small pieces of paper that had been provided by her mother from her pocketbook. Alice made large, definite, strong movements with the pencils that, at times, ran off the page and onto the rug. The therapist offered larger sheets but the mother refused these, saying that her child was too young and did not need the larger sheets. Mother physically restricted Alice to the small pieces of paper by moving her hand back onto the paper. Alice responded to the limits by switching from scribbling to making holes through the paper onto the light-colored rug. Both the mother's verbal refusal and child's actions were respected and included in the therapist's solution: The therapist found some cardboard on the back of a desk pad and put it under the small pieces of paper supplied by the mother. This action did not interfere with the hole-punching movements of the child. The hole-making was a distinct and pleasurable activity for the child.
>
> Autonomy was an important and unresolved issue in this fam-

ily. Independent action was a source of concern for all members of the family. This was illustrated in a discussion during this session of what they allowed Alice to eat. The parents were also very concerned about how she ate her food. They were uncertain about allowing her to pick food up in her fingers, or whether to continue to feed her. In the next session, Father held this child within tight limits so that she could not play freely. He enclosed her between his two legs and made them into a small circle which became her confined play area. Issues of autonomy continued to occupy play and talk for a number of family sessions.

A potential mess may be controlled, or overcontrolled, by family members, both siblings and parents, rather than by the therapist. The therapist was aware of her own strong feelings of wanting Alice to be set free. The family could not allow strong, autonomous actions, like making "dirty" holes in almost anything, but only tolerated very controlled, small pieces of paper. They had to reject the freer situation, namely the larger pieces of paper. And the Father had to define play within the area of the small circle made by his legs.

If the office has an uncarpeted, easily cleanable area, and if the therapist wishes, then washable paints, a potentially messy material, may be provided, contained within a paintbox attached to a small, low easel. If this is done, painting clothes, which are old shirts or anything that can easily cover street clothes, are a useful addition to the supplies. A specific, safe, and contained area for messes, with a playtable or an easel, is not required but is found useful by some therapists. This is a matter of personal preference.

IV. MESSES CHILDREN MAKE

Jane spontaneously initiates cleaning up by taking the cupcake plate to the nearby bathroom as Father starts on the table. (Photo 7.14)

Father finishes the job with Mother abstaining from the cleanup but looking on with pleasure. It was all so easy! The therapist also looks pleased. (Photo 7.15)

Father and the two children retrieve the M&M's that spilled as Mother holds her head! Messes were often just too much for Mother. (Photo 7.16)

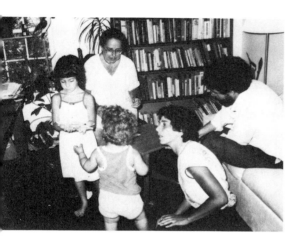

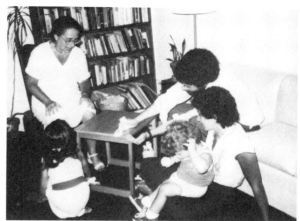

Photo 7.14

Photo 7.15

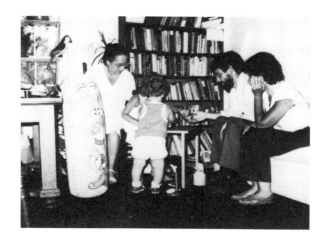

Photo 7.16

143

GOING TO THE BATHROOM: BATHROOM PLAY

After toilet training is accomplished in early childhood, interest in bathroom concerns diminishes and bodily functions in general become increasingly private and self-contained concerns. Thus, "I have to go . . . ," expressed directly and loudly, or in some other form such as wiggling or whispering into a parent's ear, may cause uneasiness in an adult therapist who is beginning his therapy experience with young children.

Older children may simply be given permission, told where the bathroom is, and possibly shown by the therapist if there are any geographic complications. We must also not forget size: Even if they can find their way easily to the toilet, young children do need help getting on and off adult-sized toilets. All this is easy to forget in the adult world of bathroom privacy. If a parent or a sibling offers help, always accept it as these are opportunities for observing parental attitudes and sibling alliances. However, a more difficult and frequently occurring situation for the therapist is when the child announces his need to go to the bathroom with someone and nobody in the family moves or responds in any way to this direct request. Should a therapist actually leave the room? This is not customary in adult therapeutic practice. A direct request to the therapist, "You take me to potty," is another unusual aspect of including younger children. Young children often see therapists as another version of a teacher or nursery school helper. The concept of making the therapy room a safe place will be tested by young children. They will find out in basic ways whether the therapist means what s/he says. Responding to a direct request to "go potty" and accompanying a young child to the toilet is often a good place to start.

Dallying in the bathroom, however, is also a way, not only of gaining special attention, but also of keeping the therapist away from the rest of the family. Additionally, there is great pleasure for the toddler in bathroom play with toilet paper, water, etc. Saying and acting on "enough" is another unusual aspect of therapeutic practice when young children are present. But saying "We have to go back now" has to be combined with respect for the toilet play needs of the toddler. Another useful way of handling repeated toilet needs is to ask for help from others in the family. The physical or action parts of bathroom doings are fairly simple, but the feelings roused in the therapist are complicated and likely to cause annoyance with a child who frequently says, "I have to go." A therapist who has had little or no experience with young children may feel reluctant when a young child sits and waits, automatically expecting to be wiped. This expectation may not be voiced in words but in an upward look from the toilet seat or by a scrunched wad of toilet paper being handed to the therapist. Pulling lots and lots of toilet paper from the roll is also fun, particularly in the presence of a therapist who does not stop the action. This is another easy test in limit setting for the knowledgeable, young-child-including family therapist.

Repeated bathroom trips in still young, but slightly older children represent a different problem. After it is clear that a toilet need has been satisfied, discussion of staying away from the session by staying out of the room should be initiated by the therapist. A typical example follows:

> Billy, nine years old, ran in and out of the family therapy room several times. Each time he announced, "I have to go." As he started out the door for the fifth time in about 15 minutes, the therapist said, "Billy, stop for a minute!" Billy looked surprised as the therapist asked, "What's up with you?" "I'm mad," Billy blurted out and launched into a tirade against his younger sibling, who had been receiving a lot of attention from other specialists about his "problems." His unspoken anger and need for attention was directed away from running out of the room, ostensibly to the toilet, and into words.

V. GOING TO THE BATHROOM: BATHROOM PLAY

In this sequence, Kenny plays in the bathroom:

He flushes the toilet. (Photo 7.17)

Here Kenny watches the water "go way." (Photo 7.18)

He looks at the water left on his hand after dipping his hand into the swirling action. This toilet play was fascinating to him and he repeated these actions until stopped by the therapist. They had been out of the room long enough! (The therapist is at the door and so cannot be seen in these pictures.) (Photo 7.19)

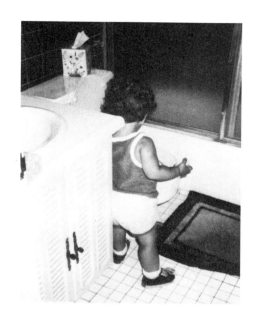

Photo 7.17

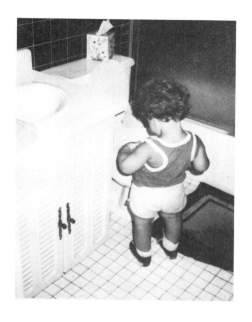

Photo 7.18

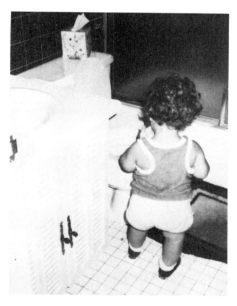

Photo 7.19

147

PICTURES: LOOK, SEE, FEEL

Abstract words, talk, and ideas occupy such a large part of the adult world. After the concrete play materials we put into our offices are used by children, what do we do then? Basically, and above all other considerations, when children make pictures or other objects, look at them directly and obviously. And don't worry! Take note of the various parts of the picture or object and comment, without asking a "Why" question. The young child doesn't know how to answer in words, "Why did you make that tree so black?" We may want to know the answer, and even have some ideas, but our thoughts are at a level of complexity that is not yet present in the young child. Simple comments like, "That's a really black tree," or, "Look at that face, it's so sad," will often elicit some verbal responses from young children. You may ask concrete questions like, "What's that?" when something is unclear. But questions starting with "Why" about drawings or other productions are to be avoided as they ask a child for an adult explanation.

Paintings and other art productions often worry therapists. They become concerned about what they – the therapists – know about "symbolic" meanings and development levels. Understanding the details of children's drawings is rarely important (Note 3). More often, the therapist may be overconcerned with meaning because s/he may not be sure how to explain or "interpret" the pictures. Interpretation per se is very rare in a family session, and only occurs when some "meaning" is very obvious:

While his parents expounded on "his" problems, Tom, age 10, painted vigorously. His five-year-old brother sat on the floor watching as Tom quickly and neatly outlined a heart with broad strokes and then poured black paint into it. Some drops of paint landed outside the edge of the heart. Tom turned these into clear, round spots connected to and coming from the heart.

The parents characterized Tom as moody, difficult, obstinate, and distant from the family. During the conversation, Tom said loudly to his younger brother, "How's that?" His brother answered, "Good." This interchange interrupted the parents' description and the therapist's attention was directed to the boys and the painting. In this instance, since it seemed so clear, the therapist made a simple interpretive comment about the picture. "That looks like a bleeding heart. But it's black. Is it a sad heart?" The parents looked surprised and Tom nodded his head in agreement.

After children complete their pictures they do many different things with them. The simplest is when they present the drawing to the therapist or to some member of the family. The child may also crumple the picture and throw it into the wastebasket or some other part of the room. The therapist must then decide whether to take the picture out during the session or rescue it afterwards. A simple comment that notices the throwing away and wonders about this, since the therapist is interested in the picture, may produce only a blank expression or some other minimal response by the child. The therapist can try to catch a picture that is being thrown and ask, as the picture is smoothed out, for permission to look at it. A caught picture is worth two in the wastebasket! If the child hands the drawing directly to a parent, then the therapist might say, "May I see it?" When a child indicates or says, "No," this is always to be respected. Other tactics may also be devised to represent interest in and appreciation of the young child's pictures. Discussion may be extended by talking about the pictures or with the pictures. The therapist not only observes drawings but the full extent of the action around the pictures in these discussions.

Sometimes children draw on both sides of the paper and consider the two sides as one communication (see Drawings 6.6 and 6.7 in Chapter 6). All kinds of variations are possible, and therapists may have to twist and turn the pictures in order to see them properly. Such freedom may seem improper to adults who, accustomed to established presentations as in a museum or art gallery, look straight ahead and stand in the right position! The therapist will have to break these adult habits when looking at young children's drawings in family sessions.

VI. PICTURES: LOOK, SEE, FEEL

Jane finishes her picture and asks the therapist for help in tearing it out of the pad. (Photo 7.20)

She decides to give it to her mother. Notice Kenny's pouting, displeased reaction as Mother delights in the gift from Jane, a smiling girl's face with a perky bow and four little hearts surrounding the picture. (Photo 7.21)

Jane throws an unfinished picture at the therapist. (Photo 7.22)

The therapist succeeds in catching it (!) and, at Jane's insistence, throws it in the wastebasket. (Photo 7.23)

Kenny tears another piece off so that he too can play. (Photo 7.24)

Kenny delightedly adds another crumpled piece of paper to the ones already thrown into the basket. Notice that in the preceding photograph Mother is watching Kenny's tearing actions with some concern. But both parents appear pleased in this photograph as he succeeds. (Photo 7.25)

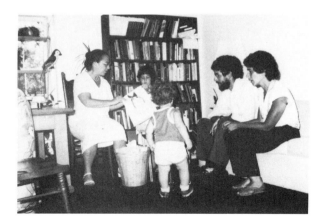

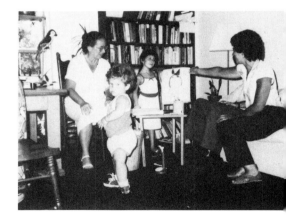

Photo 7.20   Photo

150

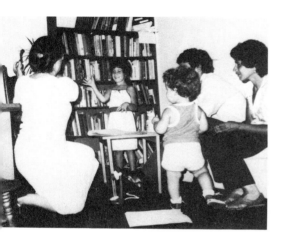

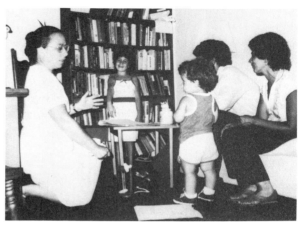

Photo 7.22

Photo 7.23

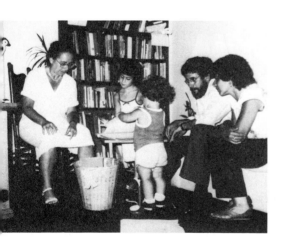

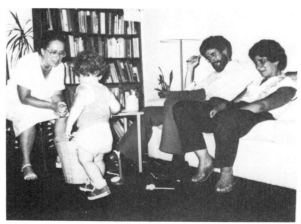

Photo 7.24

Photo 7.25

151

CELEBRATIONS: BIRTHDAYS, HOLIDAYS, AND OTHER SPECIAL OCCASIONS

> *. . . there is a significant restitutive, regenerative potential in such events as family gatherings, religious observances, feasts and festivals, weddings and births, death and the rituals of mourning. For within the context of family healing, the shared experiences come to symbolize the triumph of life over death, of pleasure over pain; in short, they are perceived as a reaffirmation of the joy of being alive.*
>
> —Nathan Ackerman, 1972, p. 440

Holidays, birthdays, and other special occasions are particularly important to young children (Note 4). They mark the calendar and the passage of time in a very concrete fashion, without the use of reading or writing. Though adults may recognize and talk about holidays and birthdays in family sessions, children recognize time, people, and feelings by remembering the celebrations, rituals, and particularly the symbols and objects connected with these events.

When children are part of family treatment, it is useful to recognize the important holidays in concrete, simple ways, for example, with candy canes or some other nonreligious marker at Christmas and Chanukah, pumpkins or marshmallow faces at Halloween, marshmallow bunnies or chocolate eggs at Easter, and recognition of other important holidays which are related to the family's ethnic or religious background. The recognition of a holiday helps establish and strengthen the therapeutic alliance, especially with children. Small children may also bring in their forms of recognition of these events, and it is important to accept their offerings. These may arrive in many forms and shapes, such as food, pictures, or other homemade presents. The family's discussions of the holidays will illustrate many aspects of their interactions. The events of the therapy session may allow experimentation with interventions and ways of communication as yet still untried at home. It is important, however, as is always the case in family therapy, for the parents not to feel outdone by the therapist. Some simple recognitions by the therapist have already been mentioned.

Birthdays deserve some special attention. It may surprise a therapist to hear a request from a youngster to have a birthday party during the family therapy session. This should be worked out jointly with the family so that birthday items are brought in mostly by the family. Candles, birthday napkins, and a cake are easy and sufficient and will not interfere with serious treatment. The celebration becomes part of family life within the therapist's office. The change from concentration on talk to eating birthday cake may elicit some questions in the mind of the therapist, such as "Is this therapy?" It may seem to the therapist that such an event is too close to actual family life. Careful concern with parents' feelings as well as serious regard of children's requests, are crucial to successfully including such occasions in treatment.

A reaction within the therapist may be that having funny Halloween faces in the office is silly! "Becoming childish" as a positive experience has been described more formally in psychoanalytic theory as a mechanism of defense, entitled "regression in the service of the ego" (Kris, 1952) (Note 5). The use of this mechanism is not only important to family therapists who work with children, but has also been discussed more broadly by Kris in relation to creativity. Creativity, though necessary, may not be readily available to therapists who shun the use of this internal psychological mechanism.

The family therapist interacts, observes, and intervenes with the child and the family during a holiday celebration within the family therapy. The recognition of holidays within a family repeats generational patterns that have been attended to faithfully and well. Families in transition, however, may have little or nothing in the way of established patterns. Frequently there is family conflict around holidays, but the pleasure may be stronger than the pain, if aided by reflection, discussion, and full family celebration.

VII. CELEBRATIONS: BIRTHDAYS, HOLIDAYS, AND OTHER SPECIAL OCCASIONS

Kenny's birthday was celebrated in a later family therapy session.

Parents watch seriously as therapist lights the candles on the birthday cup-cakes. (Photo 7.26)

But at first only Jane, Mother and the therapist blow out the candles – Kenny watches! (Photo 7.27)

The candles are relighted by the therapist and it is Kenny's turn. He is clearly pleased, Jane less so! (Photo 7.28)

Mother quickly takes the cupcake to help Kenny as Jane dives mouth-first into hers. The birthday napkins can be seen on the table. (Photo 7.29)

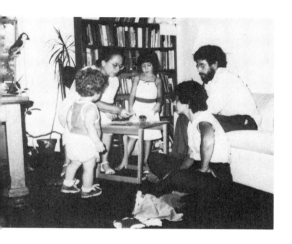

Photo 7.26

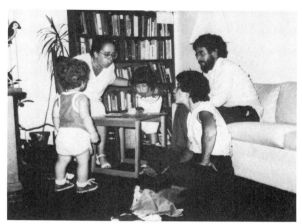

Photo 7.27

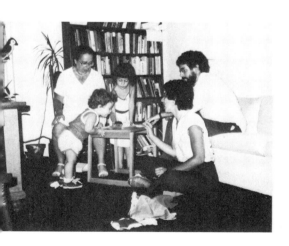

Photo 7.28

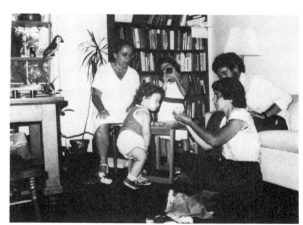

Photo 7.29

SUMMARY

In this chapter we have discussed various how-to's, including case vignettes. Photographs of actual examples of these how-to's have also been provided. The photographs that follow will provide some direct visual contact with sessions of family therapy with young children. Videotapes are even better, but are, of course, beyond the scope of this book. These how-to's are only an introduction to working with young children in family therapy. Readers who venture into this world will find their own way aided by the many tools and techniques that are already within the literature in the field of family therapy.

CHAPTER NOTES

1) Concepts of psychoanalytic growth and development make up the underlying fabric of this book. This underlying matrix is derived from the work of many but, in particular, Anna Freud, who formulated the important and useful concept of developmental lines. She discussed this extensively in an article, "The Concept of Developmental Lines: Their Diagnostic Significance." One line is of particular importance for our work in this book:

> *From Play to Work*
> . . . mothers . . . witness the first phase of the infant's play (on his own body, on the body of the mother, with cuddly toys which symbolize partly the child's own body and partly that of the mother) . . . . The child's play activity proceeds from motor play with sand and water to building, constructing, and mechanics, to role and fantasy play . . . .
> . . . Play lasts only as long as it affords pleasure; work must continue until the predetermined goal is reached.
> . . . Thus, we can understand the concept of developmental lines as an integrative one. The stages of the integrated line represent the outcome in the child or adult of both internal and external and conflictual compromise." (Freud, A. 1981a, p. 133)

2) When there is concern about a high level of activity it is useful at times to *reduce* the stimulation in the room. Toys can be put away and less material put out.
3) The developmental details of children's drawings have been studied extensively. There are a number of books that cover this special area. A short, well-written paperback volume, which also has some pictures, is: *Children's Art* by Miriam Lindstrom, 1957.
4) The quote at the beginning of this section is from Nathan Ackerman, one of a number of family therapists who sees therapeutic potential in celebrations and shared rituals, both within family therapy and family life in general. Ackerman further describes this belief about the importance of these shared experiences in his article, "The Growing Edge of Family Therapy" (Ackerman in Sager & Kaplan, 1972).

5) In a brief but specific article on young children and family therapy, Dowling and Jones (1978) are in agreement with the thesis of this volume about the frequent "dismissal" of young children from family therapy. In addition, in their discussion of countertransference, they mention the arousal of the "child within the therapist." This is of interest since this aspect is not frequently mentioned. We presented countertransference, in the discussion of reluctance and objections in an earlier chapter, as a need for the therapist to be able to be positively childish – "regression in the service of the ego" (Kris, 1952). In addition, one of their clinical descriptions includes a family with a toddler, which is also rare in the literature.

8

Finale:

"I'll Be Glad to See
All of You—
Including the Little Ones"

> *The fathers have eaten sour grapes, and the children's teeth*
> *are set on edge.*
> –Ezekiel XV 123.2 (*Oxford Dictionary of Quotations*, 1966)

> *Men deal with life as children with their play, who first misuse,*
> *then cast their toys away.*
> –William Cowper (*Oxford Dictionary of Quotations*, 1966)

The two imaginary interviews that follow will bring us back from the intricacies of the case vignettes, specific how-to's, drawings and photographs to the underlying message of this book. The first interview (1) is set in Vienna – the first "family therapy" case of Little Hans; the second (2) in Boston – an imaginary ideal case that follows the principle of this book.

1) 19 BERGASSE, VIENNA, JANUARY 1908

"Good afternoon, Dr. _____ (Little Hans's father). And, how is the (child) analysis going? You brought a picture today. . . . How interesting,

159

you drew a giraffe and your son, Hans, said, 'Draw its widdler too.' You answered, 'Draw it yourself.' He drew a short stroke and then added a bit, remarking, 'Its widdler's longer. . . . '

"I remember when your second child, Hanna, Hans's sister, was born. Hans was sleeping in your bedroom, as he had always done, until your wife started her labor. You told me some of the explanation Hans told you about the birth. He was only three and a half years old when Hanna was born. After he got sick, when he was four and three-quarters, it was so difficult to get your wife to stop "coaxing" with him (getting into bed in the morning with his mother), and allowing him to watch her in the bathroom. He was so interested in seeing her make "lumpf." Hans's analysis was aided when you enticed him to come into my consulting room (after he had refused) by telling him I had a daughter named Anna. The three of us had a good talk. . . . It was sad that such a cheerful, happy boy was suffering so, unable to go outside because he was afraid of horses, afraid that they would bite him."

2) BOSTON, MASSACHUSETTS, JULY 1982

"Hello. – Yes, your child's difficulties sound troublesome. – Yes, I'll see all of you next week. – Yes, your whole family. – What? – No, don't leave out the baby. – Yes, I know she doesn't talk yet. She's too young for that, but not for our family session. We'll discuss this more when I see all of you. – Goodbye."

In the first imaginary interview, which was based on the real case of little Hans (Freud, 1909), Hanna and Mother were not included in or after the one interview with Father, Little Hans, and Professor Freud. The second imaginary excerpt restates the message of this book.

Some years later, when "Little Hans" was asked about the psychoanalysis and treatment by his father and Freud for his horse phobia as a child, he could not remember much about it. Most therapists are very interested in follow-up and the results of treatment. Since therapists are interested in change, particularly positive change, they look to family therapy outcome research for "proof" of the benefits of their therapeutic endeavors. (The follow-up and positive "results of one family, the Roberts, have been described in Chapter 6.) I would have liked to finish this book by reporting some proof-positive results and hard data. However, outcome research on evaluation and the results of treatment are still quite uncertain, not only in regard to family therapy, but about psychotherapy in general. Family therapy has been shown in some studies to be effective, but not with great certitude (Gurman & Kniskern, 1981a).

Although an overall review of outcome research does indicate that family therapy is an effective treatment, this has not been adequately tested. The one review on this subject (Masten, 1979) does conclude that family therapy obtains positive results for children, particularly for delinquent adolescents and psychosomatically ill children:

> Among the 14 studies included in this review, only two, I felt, were controlled studies (Hardcastle, 1977; Martin, 1977). However, I did come to the conclusion that some empirical evidence does exist that family therapy is an effective treatment for children; the data from studies of adolescents are especially encouraging . . . (p. 325). A global determination of positive outcome . . . the estimated rate of improvement was 71%. (Masten, 1979, p. 330)

Improvement, however, is a very diverse matter in these studies. The author emphasizes both the methodological problems and the serious shortcomings of this research. In one of the "excluded" papers, improvement by age grouping was reported:

> Their analysis showed a somewhat higher improvement rate for *younger children*, but methodological shortcomings in this study preclude me from interpretation of age differences. (Masten, 1979, p. 331; author's emphasis)

Though simple case studies may not be regarded as convincing evidence, an interesting positive single case outcome is reported in Tiller (1978). The author specifically chose "family therapy alone" as an opportunity to assess its effectiveness without drug treatment for an eight-year-old who had a tic. Initially, other family members considered themselves "normal," as did the other staff (hospital) members. But there was "other" family trouble! Family sessions were held in a playroom and a picture produced by the identified patient is reproduced in the article. The picture figured significantly in the therapeutic work when the family wanted to stop coming and was becoming more symptomatic. In seven sessions, the tic ceased and substantial changes in whole family interactions occurred. Our conclusion to this effort is that the "hard" data so far are only promising and the one case study encouraging.

The opening chapter of this book noted that we all know what a family

161

is, or think we do, since our experience includes being born into a family, being surrounded by a family of growing children, and leaving our original families to create new household units – new families. Perhaps this familiarity has contributed to the rapid growth of family therapy as a new addition to our psychotherapeutic armamentarium, beginning in the mid-fifties. What was new or different about family therapy as a form of psychotherapy?

Family therapy is based on the premise that in selected cases, the family unit is the preferred focus of intervention to ameliorate certain discomforts, commonly called "symptoms." These discomforts may present themselves as complaints by or about a single individual who is a member of the family unit, but, nevertheless, we interpret them as signs that the whole family unit is in difficulty. Family therapy has developed and elaborated on the fundamental proposition that "the family is a unit," or stated differently, that the family treated as a whole has many advantages (Minuchin, 1974; Zilbach, 1974).

This volume has expanded upon the advantages of including young children as integral parts of the whole family unit. In particular, children can perform "critical functions" in the family therapeutic process. But, for many family therapists, the "unit," or "whole," encompasses only those family members who have reached certain prescribed ages and levels in their mental and emotional development, and who are able to express themselves "adequately on a verbal level." Inasmuch as they cannot fulfill these criteria, young, nonverbal children, and others who have limited verbal facilities, are frequently excluded from treatment. Often, only the adolescent "talkers" are considered to be eligible for inclusion in family therapy sessions. Thus, we are faced with the contradiction whereby a fundamental principle of family therapy is widely violated by its own adherents: The whole family is often *not* the unit of treatment in family therapy.

A clinically useful definition of "the family" was discussed in an earlier chapter. Although many recent structural changes have created alternative family units, families, or "household units" of some variety, these groups still perform basic family functions that are essential to the stability, growth, and development of all members, including young children. These basic family functions continue, with progressive modifications, throughout the entire family life cycle (Zilbach, 1979; 1982).

When basic functions are impaired, arrested, or even cease to function, all family members suffer. The impact on the nonverbal, younger children may seem to be less serious, because it is less apparent to adult observers, who use as their primary evidence overt, verbal statements. However, by listening with a third ear, and looking with a child-oriented eye, we can hear and see the many effects whole family disturbances have on young children.

Finally, if the assumption that there are times when the whole family is in trouble is correct, then the younger children of a troubled family must also need help. To leave children completely out of the treatment unit is to run the risk that they may remain unhelped and become a source of future trouble for their family and themselves (Bell, 1967) (Notes 1 and 2).

Thus, including the entire family, even the younger children, is essential to the family's sense of identity and to the therapist's understanding of the family's developmental history. A therapist cannot expect to fully understand a family's past history, current situation, or future hopes and fears as a family, unless s/he knows all members of the family.

Even pictorial cries for help are clear, if they are available and considered as suitable evidence. There are illustrations of several "help" messages on the frontispiece. Messages may appear in strange and obscure places. "Help" pictures have been found crumpled in wastebaskets. When family tensions were at an extreme level of intensity, one child wrote on the back of the toy box, which was against the wall of the office, "Love can keep us together."

When studious, adult family therapists review their treatment cases and evaluate progress, the question often arises, "Is the family working in treatment?" But is the content or the material of "work in treatment" only words, or does it include play, pictures, games, and photographs? Often children's play is not considered to be serious work. Work and play are often automatically contrasted and sometimes even placed in a strict order: first work, then play. As if only some kind of work entitles one to play! This is misleading, inaccurate, and inappropriate for working with families, particularly those with young children. I would like to emphasize and emphatically restate that play *is* a child's work.

Throughout this book, the importance of play, pictures and the like have been emphasized. And, though a picture may not be worth quite a thousand words, I do hope that you have really looked at the pictures and not only read the words.

CHAPTER NOTES

1) The exclusion of young children in family therapy is specifically noted in a recent review article by Levant and Haffey (1981):

> Conjoint family therapy claims to take the system as a whole in review, yet it fails to attain adequately to the smallest part – the young children. An integration of child and family therapy is recommended. . . . (p. 9)

In an earlier article, McDermott and Char emphasize the same point:

> It is our belief that with the assumption of general systems theory as the basic scheme of family therapy, there came both an indirect and a direct ejection of children from the family therapy process as they became viewed as miniature adults. (McDermott & Char, 1974, p. 425)

Thus, McDermott and Char draw a strong connection between the adoption of a theory and the "ejection" that I have termed "exclusion" of children. I have not discussed this controversial connection directly in the chapter since it deserves further consideration and research.

2) Funerals, like family therapy, often exclude young children. Bowen, who omits young children in his actual clinical practice of family therapy, has a beautiful description of including children in a most important way in funerals (Bowen, 1976 pp. 345-348).

164

Epilogue: Hopes

Writing this book has been exciting for me. My rereading of the older family therapy literature, and new reading of the more recent literature, confirmed my convictions well beyond my original expectations. Children occupy a distinct *minority* position within family therapy, i.e., that they are often excluded from treatment was very clear. Exclusion, unrecognized by the majority, is an important aspect of the experience of all minorities. I believe that the continuing and future progress of the field of family therapy may be enhanced by the elimination of exclusionary practices.

I do hope family therapists will be influenced to:

- include young children in family therapy;
- provide safety for children;
- listen with respect to children's words;
- look at children's drawings and other products;
- play with children with pleasure and understanding; and
- see the many potentially whole families that they encounter.

Although "play" is intrinsically child's work, may it become an integral and everyday part of your work as a family therapist and happily increase over the years.

Specific References to Young Children in Family Therapy

Ackerman, N. (1970). Child participation in family therapy. *Family Process, 9*, 403-410.

Bergel, E., Gass, C., & Zilbach, J. (1968). The use of play materials in conjoint therapy. Proceedings of the IVth International Congress of Group Psychotherapy. *Verlag der Weiner Medizinischen Akademie*, 4-16.

Bloch, D. A. (1976). Including the children in family therapy. In P. Guerin (Ed.), *Family therapy: Theory and practice*. New York: Gardner Press.

Chasin, R. (1981). Involving latency and preschool children in family therapy. In A. Gurman (Ed.), *Questions and answers in the practice of family therapy*, Vol. I. New York: Brunner/Mazel.

Dowling, E., & Jones, H. V. R. (1978). Small children seen and heard in family therapy. *Journal of Child Psychotherapy, 4*(4), 87-96.

Gordetsky, S., Zilbach, J., & Bennett, M. (1979, April 1). Child therapy – Its contribution to family therapy. Paper presented at the annual meeting of the American Orthopsychiatric Association.

Guttman, H. (1975). The child's participation in conjoint family therapy. *Journal of the American Academy of Child Psychiatry, 14*, 490-499.

Haley, J. (1973). Strategic therapy when a child is presented as a problem. *Journal of the American Academy of Child Psychiatry, 12*, 641-659.

Levant, R. F., & Haffey, N. A. (1981). Integration of child and family therapy. *International Journal of Family Therapy, 3*(2), 5-10.

Montalvo, B., & Haley, J. (1973). In defense of child therapy. *Family Process, 12*, 227-244.

Tiller, J. W. G. (1978). Brief family therapy for childhood tic syndrome. *Family Process, 17*, 217-223.

Villeneuve, C. (1979). The specific participation of the child in family therapy. *Journal of the American Academy of Child Psychiatry, 18*, 44-53.

Zilbach, J. (1977, November 5-6). The critical functions of the young child in family therapy. Paper presented at Symposium on the Young Child in Family Therapy. The Psychotherapy Institute and Continuing Education Program, Beth Israel Hospital and Harvard Medical School, Boston, MA.

Zilbach, J. (1982). Young children in family therapy. In A. Gurman (Ed.), *Questions and answers in the practice of family therapy*, Vol. II. New York: Brunner/Mazel, pp. 65-68.

Zilbach, J., Bergel, E., & Gass, C. (1972). The role of the young child in family therapy. In C. Sager, & H. S. Kaplan (Eds.), *Progress in group and family therapy*. New York: Brunner/Mazel.

Bibliography

Ackerman, N. W. (1938). The unity of the family. *Archives of Pediatrics*, 55, 51-62.

Ackerman, N. W. (1958). *The psychodynamics of family life*. New York: Basic Books.

Ackerman, N. W. (1966). *Treating the troubled family*. New York: Basic Books.

Ackerman, N. W. (1967). The emergence of family diagnosis and treatment: A personal view. *Psychotherapy*, Vienna, 4, 125-129.

Ackerman, N. W. (1970). Child participation in family therapy. *Family Process*, 9(4), 403-410.

Ackerman, N. W. (1972). The growing edge of family therapy. In C. Sager, & H. S. Kaplan (Eds.), *Progress in group and family therapy*. New York: Brunner/Mazel.

Ackerman, N. W., Beatman, F. L., & Sherman, S. N. (Eds.) (1956). *Expanding theory and practice in family therapy.* New York: Family Service Association of America.

Aponte, H., & Hoffman, L. (1973). The open door: A structural approach to a family with an anorectic child. *Family Process*, 12(1), 1-44.

Axline, V. M. (1947, revised 1969). *Play therapy*. New York: Ballantine Books.

Bateson, G. (1961). The biosocial integration of behavior in the schizophrenic family. In N. W. Ackerman, F. L. Beatman, & S. Sanford (Eds.), *Exploring the base for family therapy*. New York: Family Service Association of America.

Bateson, G. (1971). *Steps to an ecology of mind*. New York: Ballantine Books.

Bateson, G., Jackson, D. D., Haley, J., & Weakland, J. H. (1956) Toward a theory of schizophrenia. *Behavioral Science*, 1, 251-264.

Bateson, G., Jackson, D. D., Haley, J., & Weakland, J. H. (1963). A note on the double bind. *Family Process*, 2, 154-161.

Bell, J. E. (1961). *Family group therapy*. Public Health Monograph #64, U.S. Department of Health, Education and Welfare. Washington, D.C.: U.S. Government Printing Office.

Bell, J. E. (1967). Family group therapy – A new treatment method for children. *Family Process*, 6, 254-263.

Bergel, E. W., Gass, C., & Zilbach, J. J. (1968). The use of play materials in conjoint therapy. Proceedings of the IVth International Congress of Group Psychotherapy. *Verlag der Weiner Medizinischen Akademie*, 4-16.

Bertalanffy, von. L. V. (1968). *General systems theory*. New York: Braziller.

Bloch, D. A. (1976). Including the children in family therapy. In P. Guerin (Ed.), *Family therapy: Theory and practice*. New York: Gardner Press.

Boszormenyi-Nagy, I., & Framo, J. (Eds.) (1965). *Intensive family therapy*. New York: Harper & Row (Brunner/Mazel, 1985).

Boszormenyi-Nagy, I., & Spark, G. (1975). *Invisible loyalties*. New York: Harper & Row (Brunner/Mazel, 1984).

169

Bowen, M. (1959). Family relationships in schizophrenia. In A. Auerback (Ed.), *Schizophrenia: An integrated approach* (pp. 147-148). New York: Roland Press.

Bowen, M. (1960). A family concept of schizophrenia. In D. D. Jackson (Ed.), *The etiology of schizophrenia*. New York: Basic Books.

Bowen, M. (1976). Family reaction to death. In P. Guerin (Ed.), *Family therapy: Theory and practice*. New York: Gardner Press.

Bowen, M. (1978). *Family therapy in clinical practice*. New York: Jason Aronson.

Bowlby, J. (1949). The study and reductions of group tension in the family. *Human Relations, 2*, 123-128.

Carroll, L. (1865). *Alice's adventures in wonderland*. New York: Heritage Press, 1941.

Carroll, L. (1871). *Through the looking-glass and what Alice found there*. New York: Heritage Press, 1941.

Carter, E., & McGoldrick, M. (Eds.) (1980). *The family life cycle: A framework for family therapy*. New York: Gardner Press.

Chasin, R. (1981). Involving latency and preschool children in family therapy. In A. Gurman (Ed.), *Questions and answers in the practice of family therapy*, Vol. I (pp. 32-35). New York: Brunner/Mazel.

Degler, C. (1980). *At odds: Women and the family in America from the Revolution to the present*. New York: Oxford University Press.

Dowling, E., & Jones, H. V. R. (1978). Small children seen and heard in family therapy. *Journal of Child Psychotherapy, 4*(4), 87-96.

Entin, A. (1981). The use of photographs and family albums. In A. Gurman (Ed.), *Questions and answers in the practice of family therapy*, Vol. I (pp. 421-425). New York: Brunner/Mazel.

Erickson, G. D., & Hogan, T. P. (1976). *Family therapy: An introduction to theory and technique*. New York: Jason Aronson.

Erikson, E. (1950). *Childhood and society*. New York: W. W. Norton.

Erikson, E. (1951). Sex differences in the play configurations of preadolescents. *American Journal of Orthopsychiatry, 21*, 667-692.

Ferber, A., Mendelsohn, M., & Napier, A. (1972). *The book of family therapy*. New York: Jason Aronson.

Flugel, J. C. (1921). *The psychoanalytic study of the family*. London: Hogarth Press, 1960.

Freud, A. (1981a). The concept of developmental lines: Their diagnostic significance. *Psychoanalytic Study of the Child, 36*, 129-127.

Freud, A. (1981b). The principle task of child analysis. In *The writings of Anna Freud: Psychoanalytic psychology of normal development*, Vol. VIII, 1970-1980 (pp. 96-109). New York: International Universities Press.

Freud, S. (1905). Fragment of an analysis of a case of hysteria. In J. Strachey (Ed.), *Standard edition*, Vol. 7 (pp. 7-122). London: Hogarth Press, 1953.

Freud, S. (1908). Creative writers and daydreaming. In J. Strachey (Ed.), *Standard edition*, Vol. 9 (pp. 143-153). London: Hogarth Press, 1959.

Freud, S. (1909). Analysis of a phobia in a five year old boy. In J. Strachey (Ed.), *Standard edition*, Vol. 10 (pp. 3-153). London: Hogarth Press, 1958.

Fulweiler, C. R. (1967). No man's land. In J. Haley, & L. Hoffman (Eds.), *Techniques of family therapy*. New York: Basic Books.

Funk & Wagnall (1980). *Standard dictionary*. New York: Lippincott & Crowell.

Gass, C., Bergel, E. W., & Zilbach, J. J. (1968). Including younger children in family therapy. Unpublished manuscript.

Gordetsky, S., Zilbach, J. J., & Bennett, M. (1979, April 1). Child therapy – Its contribution to family therapy. Paper presented at the Annual Meeting of the American Orthopsychiatric Association.

Gordetsky, S., Zilbach, J. J., Fishman, C., Johnson, N., & Bennett, M. (1984, April). Family therapy training – Are we remembering the children? Panel presentation at the Annual Meeting of the American Orthopsychiatric Association, Toronto, Canada.

Guerin, P. J. (Ed.) (1976). *Family therapy: Theory and practice.* New York: Gardner Press.

Guerin, P. J. (1976). Family therapy: The first twenty-five years. In P. J. Guerin (Ed.), *Family therapy: Theory and practice.* New York: Gardner Press.

Guntrip, H. (1971). *Psychoanalytic theory, therapy, and the self* (p. 3). New York: Basic Books.

Gurman, A. S. (Ed.) (1981). *Questions and answers in the practice of family therapy,* Vol. I. New York: Brunner/Mazel.

Gurman, A. S. (Ed.) (1982). *Questions and answers in the practice of family therapy,* Vol. II. New York: Brunner/Mazel.

Gurman, A. S., & Kniskern, D. P. (1978a). Deterioration in marital and family therapy: Empirical clinical and conceptual issues. *Family Process, 17,* 3–20.

Gurman, A. S., & Kniskern, D. P. (1978b). Research on marital and family therapy: Progress, perspective and prospect. In S. Garfield, & A. Bergin (Eds.), *Handbook of psychotherapy and behavior change.* New York: Wiley.

Gurman, A. S., & Kniskern, D. P. (1981a). Family therapy outcome research: Knowns and unknowns. In A. S. Gurman, & D. P. Kniskern (Eds.), *Handbook of family therapy,* Vol. I. New York: Brunner/Mazel.

Gurman, A. S., & Kniskern, D. P. (1981b). *Handbook of family therapy.* New York: Brunner/Mazel.

Guttman, H. A. (1975). The child's participation in conjoint family therapy. *Journal of the American Academy of Child Psychiatry, 14,* 490–499.

Guttman, H. A. (1983). La thérapie familiale auprès de jeunes enfants. *Santé Mentale du Quebec, 8,* 134–139.

Haley, J. (1957). The family of the schizophrenic: A model system. In G. D. Erickson & T. P. Hogan (Eds.), *Family therapy: An introduction to theory and technique* (pp. 357–374). New York: Jason Aronson, 1976.

Haley, J. (1973). Strategic therapy when a child is presented as a problem. *Journal of the American Academy of Child Psychiatry, 12,* 641–659.

Haley, J., & Hoffman, L. (Eds.) (1967). *Techniques of family therapy.* New York: Basic Books.

Hardcastle, V. R. (1977). A mother-child, multiple-family, counseling program procedures and results. *Family Process, 16,* 67–74.

Heard, D. (1978). Keith: A case study of structural family therapy. *Family Process, 17,* 339–356.

Hoffman, L. (1976). Breaking the homeostatic cycle. In P. J. Guerin (Ed.), *Family therapy: Theory and practice* (pp. 501–519). New York: Gardner Press.

Hoffman, L. (1981). *Foundations of family therapy.* New York: Basic Books.

Jackson, D. D. (1957). The question of family homeostasis. *Psychiatry Quarterly Supplement, 31,* 79–90. Reprinted in: *International Journal of Family Therapy,* 1981, *3*(1), 5–16.

Keith, D. V., & Whitaker, C. A. (1967). The divorce labyrinth. In P. Papp (Ed.), *Family therapy: Full-length case studies* (pp. 117–133). New York: Gardner.

Klein, M. (1932). *The psychoanalysis of children.* London: Hogarth Press.

Kohut, H. (1971). *The analysis of the self.* New York: International Universities Press.

Kohut, H. (1977). *The restoration of the self.* New York: International Universities Press.

Kramer, C. (1981). *Becoming a family therapist.* New York: Human Services Press.

Kris, E. (1952). *Psychoanalytic explorations in art.* New York: International Universities Press.

Levant, R. F., & Haffey, N. A. (1981). Integration of child and family therapy. *International Journal of Family Therapy, 3*(2), 5–10.

Lidz, T. (1958). Schizophrenia and the family. *Psychiatry, 21,* 21–27.

171

Lidz, T. (1963). *The family and human adaptation.* New York: International Universities Press.

Lidz, T., Cornelison, A., Fleck, S., & Terry, D. (1957). The intrafamilial environment of schizophrenic patients. II: Marital schism and marital skew. *American Journal of Psychiatry, 114,* 241-248.

Lindstrom, M. (1957). *Children's art: A study of normal development in children's modes of visualization.* Berkeley and Los Angeles: University of California Press.

Martin, B. (1977). Brief family intervention: Effectiveness and importance of including the father. *General Consulting Clinical Psychology, 45,* 1002-1010.

Masten, A. S. (1979). Family therapy as a treatment for children: A critical review of outcome research. *Family Process, 18*(3), 323-336.

McDermott, J. F., & Char, W. F. (1974). The undeclared war between child and family therapy. *Journal of the American Academy of Child Psychiatry, 13*(3), 422-436.

Midelfort, C. F. (1957). *The family in psychotherapy.* New York: McGraw-Hill.

Miller, J. G. (1969). Living systems: Basic concepts. In W. Gray, F. Duhl, & N. Rizzo (Eds.), *General systems theory and practice.* Boston: Little, Brown.

Minuchin, S. (1974). *Families and family therapy.* Cambridge, MA: Harvard University Press.

Mishler, E., & Waxler, N. (1968). *Interaction in families: An experimental study of family processes and schizophrenia.* New York: Wiley & Sons.

Montalvo, B., & Haley, J. (1973). In defense of child therapy. *Family Process, 12,* 227-244.

Murdock, G. P. (1949). *Social structure.* Glencoe, IL: Free Press.

Napier, A. V. (1977). Follow-up to divorce labyrinth. In P. Papp (Ed.), *Family therapy: Full-length case studies* (pp. 133-143). New York: Gardner.

Oxford Dictionary of Quotations (2nd ed.) (1966). London: Oxford University Press.

Papp, P. (Ed.) (1977). *Family therapy: Full-length case studies.* New York: Gardner.

Parsons, T., & Bales, R. F. (1955). *Family: Socialization and interaction process.* Glencoe, IL: Free Press.

Piaget, J. (1951). *Play, dreams and imitation in childhood.* New York: Norton.

Piaget, J. (1952). *Origins of intelligence.* New York: International Universities Press.

Piaget, J. (1954). *Construction of reality in the child.* New York: Basic Books.

Phillips, C. E. *Toward a theory of marriage and family counseling: Systems eclecticism.* Unpublished manuscript.

Phillips, C. E. (1980). Notes on system theory. Unpublished manuscript.

Riskin, J. (1964). Family interaction scales. *Archives of General Psychiatry, 11,* 484-494.

Sager, C. J., & Kaplan, H. S. (1972). *Progress in group and family therapy.* New York: Brunner/Mazel.

Satir, V. W. (1964). *Conjoint family therapy.* Palo Alto: Science & Behavior Books.

Serrano, A. C. (1979). A child-centered family diagnostic interview. In J. Call (Ed.), *Basic handbook of child psychiatry,* Vol. I (pp. 624-630). New York: Basic Books.

Snyder, M. H. (1979). Jennifer. In *Enough.* San Luis Obispo, CA: Solo Press.

Villeneuve, C. (1979). The specific participation of the child in family therapy. *Journal of the American Academy of Child Psychiatry, 18,* 44-53.

Weakland, J. (1960). The double-bind hypothesis of schizophrenia and three party interaction. In D. D. Jackson (Ed.), *The etiology of schizophrenia* (p. 374). New York: Basic Books.

Webster, N. (1962). *Webster's new world dictionary, college edition.* New York: World.

Webster, N. (1979). *Webster's deluxe unabridged dictionary.* New York: Simon & Schuster.

Whitaker, C. (1967). The growing edge – An interview with Carl Whitaker. In J. Haley, & L. Hoffman (Eds.), *Techniques of family therapy.* New York: Basic Books.

Whitaker, C. (1982). *From psyche to system: The evolving therapy of Carl Whitaker.* Neill, J. R. & Kniskern, D. P. (Eds.), New York: Guilford Press.

Whitaker, C., & Keith, D. V. (1981). Symbolic-experiential family therapy. In A. Gurman, & D. Kniskern (Eds.), *Handbook of family therapy* (pp. 187-226). New York: Brunner/Mazel.

Winnicott, D. W. (1971a). *Playing and reality*. New York: Basic Books.

Winnicott, D. W. (1971b). *Therapeutic consultation in child psychiatry*. New York: Basic Books.

Wynne, L. (1965). Some indications and contraindications for exploratory family therapy. In I. Boszormenyi-Nagy, & J. L. Framo (Eds.), *Intensive family therapy* (pp. 289-322). New York: Harper & Row.

Wynne, L. C., Ryckoff, M., Day, J., & Hirsch, S. K. (1958). Psuedomutuality in the family relations of schizophrenics. *Psychiatry, 21*, 205-220.

Zilbach, J. J. (1968). Family development. In J. Marmor (Ed.), *Modern psychoanalysis* (pp. 355-386). New York: Basic Books.

Zilbach, J. J. (1974). The family in family therapy. *Journal of the American Academy of Child Psychiatry, 13*(3), 459-467.

Zilbach, J. J. (1977, November 5-6). The critical functions of the young child in family therapy. Paper presented at Symposium on the Young Child in Family Therapy. The Psychotherapy Institute and Continuing Education Program, Beth Israel Hospital, Harvard Medical School, Boston, MA.

Zilbach, J. J. (1979). Family development and familial factors in etiology. In J. Noshpitz, et al. (Eds.), *Basic handbook of child psychiatry*, Vol. II (pp. 62-87). New York: Basic Books.

Zilbach, J. J. (1982). Separation: A family developmental process of midlife years. In C. Nadelson, & M. Notman (Eds.), *The woman patient*, Vol 2. New York: Plenum Press.

Zilbach, J. J. (1982). Young children in family therapy. In A. Gurman (Ed.), *Questions and answers in the practice of family therapy*, Vol. II. New York: Brunner/Mazel.

Zilbach, J. J., Bergel, E. W., & Gass, C. (1968). The family life cycle: Some developmental considerations. Proceedings of the IVth International Congress of Group Psychotherapy. *Verlag der Weiner Medizinischen Akademie*, Vienna, pp. 157-162.

Zilbach, J. J., Bergel, E. W., & Gass, C. (1972). The role of the young child in family therapy. In C. J. Sager, & H. S. Kaplan (Eds.), *Progress in group and family therapy* (pp. 385-400). New York: Brunner/Mazel.

Index

Abandonment, 104, 108
Ackerman, N. W., 26-28, 35, 41-
    42, 44, 152
Adolescence, 31, 161-162, *see also*
    Children
Aggression, 120, 135, 137
Alcoholism, 78
Alliances, 64
   therapeutic, 52-53, 152
Anger, 116, 121, 136
Anxiety, 17, 19-20, 90, 98, 121
Aponte, H., 44
Artwork, *see* Pictures
Autonomy, 140-141
Axline, V. M., 14

Bales, R. F., 8
Bateson, G., 27, 29-30
Bathroom play, 144-147
Bell, J. E., 26, 163
Bergel, E. W., 35, 45
Bertalanffy, von L. V., 29
Birthdays, 152-155
Bloch, D. A., 28, 35, 42
Brown, D., 89-123
Boundaries, 44
Bowen, M., 41, 164
Bowlby, J., 26

Carter, E., 8
Celebrations, 152-155
Char, W. F., 2, 163-164
Child abuse, 52
Child development, 131, 136
Child psychiatry, 3

Children, *see also* Adolescence; Par-
    ents; Play
  as allies and co-therapists, 52-53,
    60, 76-80
  autonomy and, 140-141
  bathroom play and, 144-147
  drive for self-expression, 42
  early detection of problems and,
    53-55, 62, 80-84
  equipment for, 131-136
  exclusion from family therapy, 11-
    12, 20-23, 37, 43, 66-68,
    163-165
  as identified patient, 45, 51
  messages about themselves, 114-
    123
  messes and, 140-143
  secrets and, 45, 66-67, 76, 137
  structural family therapy and, 31-33
  as symptom bearers, 51, 71-76
  view of child/parent relationship,
    106-114
  view of family therapy, 91-93
  view of separation and divorce, 93-
    106
Communication, double-bind, 30-31
Countertransference, 157
Creativity, 15-16, 153

Degler, C., 5
Delinquents, 161
Depression, 60, 74, 110
  severe childhood, 82, 84
Divorce, case study, 90-91, 93-106
Double-bind communication, 30-31

Dowling, E., 157
Drawings, *see* Pictures

Ego, 12, 15, 153, 157
Emptiness, 78, 104
Encopresis, 96, 98, 110
Enuresis, 74
Equipment, 131-136
  dealing with messes, 140-143
  parents' reaction to, 136-139
Erickson, G. D., 26-27
Erikson, E., 15
Executive subsystem, 32
Eye contact, 126, 130

Family
  definition of, 5-6, 162
  development, 6-8, 38-39, 55, *see
    also* Family life cycle
  homeostasis, 29-30, 36-37
  life cycle, 7-8, 55, *see also* Family
    development
Family system, 9
Family systems theory, 29-30, 37
Family therapy, 2-3, *see also* Thera-
    pists
  definition of, 8
  effectiveness of, 160-161
  exclusion of children from, 11-12,
    20-23, 37, 43, 66-68, 163-
    165
  function of children in
    as allies and co-therapists, 52-53,
      60, 76-80
    as symptom-bearers, 51, 71-76
    early problem detection and, 53-
      55, 62, 80-84
  functions of play in, 17-20
  goals for, 38
  history, 26
  playing with children in, 14
  structural, 31-33
  techniques
    bathroom play, 144-147
    dealing with messes, 140-143
    equipment for children, 131-136
    explaining purpose of sessions,
      130
    recognition of special occasions,
      152-155
    saying hello to children, 126-131

using artwork, 148-152
whole family as the unit of treat-
  ment, 162-163
whole family interactions and, 55-
  56, 64, 84-88
Fears, 54, 120
Freud, A., 11, 15, 131, 156
Freud, S., 15, 16, 46, 160
Fulweiler, C. R., 31, 36-37, 43
Funerals, 164

Gass, C., 35, 45
General systems theory, 29, 164
Gordetsky, S., 71-88, 89-124
Guerin, P. J., 27, 33
Gurman, A. S., 27, 34, 45, 160
Guttman, H. A., 44-45

Haffey, N. A., 163
Haley, J., 27, 29-30, 33, 36-40,
  43-44
Hardcastle, V. R., 161
Heard, D., 47
Hillcrest Family Series film, 41
Hoffman, L., 33, 36-40, 44, 46
Hogan, T. P., 26-27
Holidays, 152-155
Homeostasis, 29-30, 36-37
Hostility, 56

Identified patient, 51, 130
Inhibitions, 137
Intergenerational family problems, 54

Jackson, D. D., 27, 29, 36, 38, 41
Jones, H. V. R., 157
Judge Baker Guidance Center, 2-3

Kaplan, H. S., 27, 156
Keith, D. V., 35
Klein, M., 14
Kniskern, D. P., 27, 34, 160
Kohut, H., 42
Kris, E., 153, 157

Learning problems, 51
Levant, R. F., 163
Life cycle, 7-8, 55, *see also* Family
  life cycle
Limit setting, 136, 145
Lindstrom, M., 156

Loneliness, 78

Martin, B., 161
Masten, A. S., 161
McDermott, J. F., 2, 163-164
McGoldrick, M., 8
Miller, J. B., 29
Minuchin, S., 9, 31-33, 162
Mishler, E., 31
Montalvo, B., 33, 43-44
Murdock, G. P., 9

Napier, A. V., 35
Neglect, 78, 84

Omnipotence, 34

Paints, 141, *see also* Pictures
Papp, P., 36, 40, 53
Parents, 136-139, *see also* Children
    objections to including children in
        therapy, 67
Parsons, T., 8
Phillips, C. E., 9, 29
Phobias, 54
Piaget, J., 16
Pictures, 74-75, 82-84, 86, 156
    cries for help, 163
    of children's messages about them-
        selves, 114-123
    of family treatment during divorce,
        89-123
    techniques for using, 148-152
Play, 11-23, 89-90, 109, 156, *see
    also* Children
    as a way of providing insights, 74-
        75
    in the bathroom, 144-147
    as child's work, 163, 165
    creativity and, 15-16
    dealing with messes, 140-143
    definition of, 43
    equipment for children, 131-136
    in family therapy, 17-20
    as a mirror of family action, 43-44
    parents' reactions to, 136-139
    real/make believe, 45
    structural family therapy and, 32-33
    therapist as playful, 42-43
    therapist's resistance to, 20-22
    value of, 12-14

Whitaker's work and, 34-35, 39-40
    work and, 15
Play therapy, 4, 14
Play-battling, 34-35

Regression, 12, 104, 153, 157
Resistance, 66-67, 137
    to continuing therapy, 78-79
Role modeling, 55

Sager, C. J., 27, 156
Satir, V. W., 26-29, 36-38
Schizophrenia, 30-31
School problems, 51
Secrets, 45, 66-67, 76, 137
Self-derogation, 116
Self-esteem, 98, 121
Separation, 54
Serrano, A. C., 45-46
Sibling subsystem, 32
Special occasions, 152-155
Squiggle game, 14
Structural family therapy, 31-33
Supplies, 131-136
    dealing with messes, 140-143
    parents' reactions to, 136-139
Symptom-bearers, 51
Systems theory, 29-30, 164

Therapeutic alliance, 52-53, 152
Therapists, *see also* Family therapy
    objections to including children in
        therapy, 66-67, 153, 157
    play experiences and, 20-22, 137
    preference in age of clients, 41
    use of self, 42
Tiller, J. W. G., 161
Toys, 131-136
    dealing with messes, 140-143
    parents' reactions to, 136-139

Villeneuve, C., 44

Waxler, N., 31
Weakland, J., 29, 31
Whitaker, C., 33-35, 36, 39-41, 53
Winnicott, D. W., 11, 14, 42
Withdrawal, 62

Zilbach, J. J., 6, 8, 30, 35, 39, 45-
    46, 69, 162